November 6th 2015

Dear diary,

There are two lines! Two lines! I'm going to be a mummy again! Overwhelmed, excited, shocked, nervous … I'm so happy that I have this precious little life growing inside me. I feel so lucky to have been blessed with another bundle of joy. Children bring me so much happiness and I cannot wait to see what this little bean brings to our family.

Cora and Maisie are 4 on January 19th – they are going to be such amazing big sisters. They're two of the most loving little beings I have ever known; and I'm not just saying this because they're mine. There are no words to describe this feeling. I just want to shout it from the rooftops already! Chris is going to be such an amazing daddy to this baby; his first baby. And I'm sure that Jake will be happy for our little girls in their new journey of becoming big sisters. There are so many emotions running through my mind:
When do I tell people?
When do I tell the girls?
Do I get excited now or wait until we are 'safe'?
Do I book an early scan for reassurance?
Do we need to move in to a bigger house?
I wonder if this bean is going to be another girl or will I have a son?

I need to calm down! Eek.

November 11th 2015.

Dear Diary,

So, I'm pathetic at keeping secrets that are my own. I can be trusted with anyone's secrets; but as soon as I have something happen in my life I NEED to share it with those close to me. I've told pretty much everyone I know. Chris OBVIOUSLY knows that he's going to be a daddy. He is nervous, but he's looking forward to it.

My dad and step-mum know, my sisters and their partners know, my closest friends know, Chris' parents know, Chris' brother knows … I can't wait to tell the girls and see their reaction. We have an early scan in December just to check on baby and make sure he/she/they (I HAVE had twins before) are growing and developing okay. It's booked for December 6th (I think) at a private clinic. I can't wait to see that little flickering heartbeat for the first time.

November 27th 2015.

Dear diary,

Morning sickness seems to have made it's dreaded appearance today; aside from that, feeling pretty good. I'm not sure if I'm just imagining things, but I seem to have a bump appear from no where. With me having twins, though, my womb is fully aware of what it's supposed to do. Also, fully capable of expanding to fit TWO babies. So, yeah, nervous about how much of a chub this little bean is going to be.

I already REALLY want to know what we're being blessed with. I know that it really doesn't matter in the grand scheme of things, but it's always nice to prepare and start window shopping for a little girl or boy.

My gut instinct is telling me that we're having a little boy this time. I couldn't tell you why; it's just that everything about this pregnancy feels 'different' to when I was pregnant with Cora and Maisie. BUT maybe that's just because I'm probably carrying just the one baby this time, not twins? Who knows … Only time will tell, I suppose. But I'm definitely looking in to booking an early gender scan.

November 28th 2015.

Dear Diary,

So, I was DEFINITELY wrong about our scan date. Turns out it was today! Anyway, we saw our little bean today for the first time! YUP, just the one! He/she is growing and developing perfectly. This just made it so much more real, seeing that teeny flickering heartbeat on the screen.

Chris seemed to enjoy it, though I think it made it a little more real that he's actually becoming a daddy now. His first little boy or girl. I'm excited for him. He really will make a great daddy – he's the one who becomes every child's Godfather. He genuinely is such a natural with children.

We have an estimated due date of July 12th, 2016. Obviously, that could possibly change at our 12 weeks dating scan, which will be much more accurate than the one we had today. I'm looking forward to having a Summer baby this time around. I think I'm going to tell Cora and Maisie tomorrow when they get home from their daddy's house. I'm reassured that I have a fantastic support network around me if (God forbid) anything happen to this baby. But, I'm sure that will not be the case. Things like that don't happen to people like me, right?

Little bean had such a strong, healthy heartbeat. I already know that he/she is going to be a fighter. We booked in today for an early gender scan. We will find out February 7th if our precious baby is a boy or a girl. I cannot wait.

November 29th 2016.

Dear Diary,

I told the girls today that they're going to be big sisters. They are SO excited! I had a lot of questions about where baby is going to sleep, if baby is a boy or a girl, when baby is going to arrive, if they can help choose his/her name …

Cora really wants a little sister. She said she will want her to be called Rapunzel and she will paint her toe nails and do her hair. Maisie really wants a little brother, which is understandable because she's a real Tomboy at heart and would want to join him playing with cars and climbing trees. She said she will want him to be called Stuart, and they will play together all the time.

I tried my best to explain what this means for our little family. I tried my best to explain that this baby doesn't have the same daddy as they do; but they don't care. They are just over the moon to be becoming big sisters. I know they'll make the best ones, they really will. I cannot wait to watch them grow and play and learn as siblings; all three of them.

December 11th 2016.

Dear Diary,

I just couldn't hold it together anymore. This evening I made it public that Chris and I are expecting our first baby together, and the girls are expecting their first sibling. We have had nothing but good, supportive comments. It reassures me knowing we are surrounded by people that love and care about us.

After such an awful year with Maisie's hospital stay after her 2 hour long fit and 7 day long coma, followed by her diagnosis of Porencephaly & Epilepsy, and then Grandma Lilian passing away days later; I think the good news of a new family member was welcome news. It's needed. This little bean is now our hope for a better year next year.

Roll on Summer!

December 25th 2015.

Dear Diary,

Obviously, it's Christmas day. I cannot begin to explain how much I love this day. It makes me so happy seeing Cora and Maisie so happy. It's going to be even better next year, with three little people to enjoy. It will obviously be more expensive! But definitely more fun.

We have our dating scan on the 6th of January, too. Something else to look forward to. Not much to say today, I just wanted to share how much I am looking forward to watching 2 become 3, 4 become 5, in just 7 months. Eek!

January 6th 2016.

Dear Diary,

Happy New Year! We had our dating scan today. Still, just the one baby (phew!), growing very well. He/she still has a perfecty strong heartbeat and is developing great. I am 14 weeks and 1 day. 14 weeks down, 26 to go. This means our due date has been brought forward to the 7th of July! (Insert mahooooosive smiley face here).

This pregnancy seems to be flying by compared to my pregnancy with the twins. With them, it seemed to go on forever. Whether it's just because I was more apprehensive and nervous back then, I don't know.

Everything about this pregnancy seems different. I couldn't tell you why. I'm thinking it's probably because it's just one baby this time, or possibly a boy. Who knows? I'm looking forward to finding out though. 4 weeks to go and we will see what I'm growing this time!

January 19th 2016.

Dear Diary,

It's Maisie and Cora's 4th birthday today. We haven't done much for their birthday. I ended up in hospital this afternoon with a bleed. I was given an emergency scan to see what was going on – turns out I have a couple of ovarian cysts and one of them has burst, hence the bleeding. I was also told I have a low-lying placenta which could mean I may have to have a non-optional repeat cesaerean as opposed to being able to delivery naturally. I don't think I'm overly bothered either way, as long as baby gets here safe and sound that's all that matters to me.

Having the bleed really scared me. It's the first time during my pregnancy that I actually considered something could be going wrong. I am SO thankful it was just a scare and that baby is okay. I've been told to relax now, that our chances of losing this baby are less than 1% at this stage and I shouldn't be worrying.

Massive weight off my mind. Roll on next month when we get to give our baby a name! Still pretty certain I'm having a little boy, though.

February 7th 2016.

Dear Diary,

I was right ... as usual.

We are having a little BOY! I'm SO happy!

I would have been happy either way, but knowing that I'm getting a son and that, after this baby my family will be complete is amazing. There are no words to describe this happiness. I can start shopping for baby clothes and we can have a look properly at what we want to call him. Chris likes 'different' names, whereas I'm more traditional. So I'm not sure where we are going to go with this one. So far, on our list, we have:

- Lennox
- Zander
- Phoenix
- Oliver
- George

Such a long list, eh?! And I'm not sure I even like any of those names. They're just ones I would 'put up with' ... With the girls, their names just jumped off the page at me and I knew instantly. I can see this baby being born with no name.

February 14th 2016.

Dear Diary,

Chris is away for the weekend in Amsterdam with his friends. I hope he's having a great time – he seems to be anyway. He text me this morning letting me know that he has bought our little boy a baby grow from a shop over there. Not going to lie, I'm a tad nervous about what he's going to come home with. He's a man, after all. And Amsterdam is, you know ... well, Amsterdam.

I just hope whatever he has bought our little boy was purchased outside of the Red Light District! We will see, he's home late tonight, around midnight (I think).

February 19th 2016.

Dear Diary,

The baby grow wasn't as bad as I thought it would be. Admittedly (probably shamefully) it's kinda cute. It's a jersey style baby grow. Chris was super proud of himself for purchasing his first baby item. He probably won't be enjoying it as much when I start dragging him round shopping centres next weekend.

We had our 20 weeks scan yesterday. It went swimmingly. Baby boy is growing absolutely fine. He has all of his organs, they're all in perfect condition. There is NOTHING at all on his brain, which was a big concern of mine with Maisie's Porencephalic Cysts. It's just getting more 'real' by the day that this little boy is ours and he will be coming home with us. We are half way there now. I can't believe how time is flying by.

We seem to have expanded our list of possible names, but I'm still not sure if I even like any of them that much. Here they are:

- Hugo
- Phoenix
- Lennox
- George
- Louie
- Xander
- Cohen
- Miles
- Lucas

Meh. We will see. I'm hoping one just 'jumps out' at me, as they did with the girls. Then when it does, I'll just have to coax Chris in to agreeing with me.

March 2nd 2015.

OTIS! The name just fits! His name is Otis. I don't care if Chris likes it or not. I'm going to suggest it to him tonight. I would have done already but I'm worried he will turn it down, and it's the only name I really, really like. In fact, you could say I love it.

I'm terribly neurotic when it comes to baby names. I HAD to have the girls' names ready chosen well before they were born, and I'm the same with my little boy – I feel like it helps me bond with the baby growing within me. I prefer being able to talk to them with their name as opposed to calling them 'baby' … It just makes them seem more 'real' and helps them become a little person. It's also nice to feel them grow around that name. I already know that this little mister is going to be stubborn and cheeky. I can tell by the way he insists on keeping me up all night kicking, and how he doesn't like for me to put my hand on my tummy (he always kicks me off).

March 13th 2016.

Dear Dairy,

Last night was scary. I had an ambulance call out and bring me to hospital (baby is fine, it's me that's the problem). I started getting really bad blurred vision, I couldn't speak properly, the right hand side of my body started going numb and I was feeling really sick.

When the ambulance arrived my blood pressure and heart rate were both sky high. They assumed pre-eclampsia and brought me in to Resus at the hospital's A&E. I feel a little better today, the sickness seems to be wearing off, but the numbness is still here. I cannot use my right hand at all. I have no strength in it to grip. It's frustrating but I'm sure I will be okay.

I have an MRI today on my brain to make sure everything is okay. I'm nervous but I've been told that it won't affect the baby in any way, which is obviously my main concern, so that's good.

April 3rd 2016.

Dear Diary,

I know it's been a while. I haven't really felt up to talking over the last few weeks. I got discharged from hospital yesterday. The numbness has finally started wearing off but it hasn't gone completely. The sickness ended up getting worse while I was hospitalised and it got to the point where I couldn't even stomach water. My MRI came back clear, they're putting the lasting numbness and blurred vision down to blood vessel constriction in my head and around my sinuses, as well as migraines. Unusual, for me, as I suffer from migraines regularly and have never had one like that before.

I was moved to a maternity hospital so the midwives could keep a good eye on baby while I was being treated. He's fine, I'm doing fine, and we're home. Now I can focus on getting better, I can start shopping for this baby and I can spend some much needed quality time with Cora and Maisie.

April 12th 2016.

Dear Diary,

I was 27 weeks on Friday. Today is Tuesday. I'm scared. I was admitted to hospital today with substantial bleeding and suspected pre-term labour. I've been here before with the girls and I can't say I'm the least bit excited about the next few days while they work to stop this.

I have been examined and I'm 2cm dilated. The bleeding is still going strong though, and so is the pain. I'm contracting every 6-7 minutes for over a minute. The good news is that I haven't dilated any more since admission; the bad news is that NOTHING is stopping this pain and it really hurts!

Chris brought me a teddy today that he bought off baby for me for Mother's Day. Better late than never I suppose! It's cute though. It's a little kangaroo with a baby roo in it's pouch. It's also coming in handy to squeeze every time I get a pain. They still aren't letting up.

May 9th 2016.

Dear Diary,

I know I'm neglecting you. It's been a whole month since I even opened you. But I needed this time to myself. It's been a struggle. Both me and baby, who we have named Otis, have been fighting real hard.

My constant contracting (every 3-5 minutes for over 3 weeks) finally eased off last week, and I was discharged from hospital today. I ended up having to have surgery to fit a Nephrostomy Tube in to my kidney. It's nothing new to me – I had one during my pregnancy with the girls, too. It's basically a tube placed in to the kidney that protrudes out of the back and goes in to a bag. This bag collects the urine that my kidney cannot release, due to blocked tubes. I had it done without anaesthetic, but I was informed it'd be less dangerous for Otis that way. My little boy comes first so I didn't give it a second thought.

I'm shattered, I really am. Everything appears to be okay with Otis. We had a scan while we were in hospital and he's still developing perfectly, he's just growing a little slow. But that's okay; they've said it's nothing to worry about. All of his organs are in good, working order with no signs of a single problem.

We have been told to return for a growth scan on the 17th May, just to make sure baby is still growing (even if slowly). I can't wait to see him again.

May 15th 2016.

Dear Diary,

I was readmitted to hospital today. I have an infection in my kidney and the tube has become blocked and calcified so it needs removing and replacing. It's being done tomorrow.

Otis has been super active of late. He never stops moving and kicking. I love it. I keep telling Chris that he's going to become a ballet dancer; he's insistent on footballer; but I know these kicks are definitely dancer's kicks.

Otis can be whatever he wants to be, as long as he's happy and healthy. Both Chris and I couldn't careless if he wants to do a sport that is typically seen as a feminine sport, as long as he enjoys it.

May 16th 2016.

Dear Diary,

Had the neph tube replaced today. Thank God that's over with! Instant relief.

May 17th 2016.

Dear Diary,

I'm terrified. I cannot put in to words this feeling of dread I carry in my heart right now. We had a growth scan done today. They have found a growth on our little boy's brain and no one can tell us what it is just yet. We have to have a repeat scan on Thursday with a specialist consultant to decide what to do from here, and for her to give us a bigger insight on what this 'uniform mass' could possibly be.

It is 3cm in size.

How can this be happening?

We had a scan just 3 weeks ago and everything was perfectly fine. There wasn't so much as a millimetre of growth anywhere on his body, how can he now have a decent sized mass growing on his poor little brain?! I can't say I'm excited for Thursday in the least. Devastated.

May 20th 2016.

Dear Diary,

This cannot be happening. The growth on Otis' brain has grown. It's grown. Not only has it grown, it's doubled in size. Half of his poor brain is now engulfed by what they think is a brain tumour. This cannot be happening. Not to me, not to us. Things like this don't happen to people like us, right?

The consultant in charge today has insisted that I be discharged from this hospital today and we are to go to a more specialist hospital on Monday for a more in depth ultrasound scan and to see a paediatric neurologist.

May 23rd 2016.

Dear Diary,

How quickly things can change, eh?

We travelled just over two hours today to have an ultrasound with the specialist doctors. We arrived at 2:30pm for our appointment and we have JUST got home – it's 10:45pm. So, as you can imagine, today didn't go too well.

After the ultrasound we sat down with the doctor who told us that I need an urgent MRI on Otis' brain. It's been booked for tomorrow. I don't feel like talking much this eve. I'll explain more tomorrow.

May 24th 2016

Dear Diary,

We had the MRI today and were sent home to wait 3-5 days for our results. I'll explain more now about why the urgent MRI was ordered after our appointment yesterday.

Our little boy's brain is riddled in tumour and haemorraghes. Over half of his brain is engulfed by a tumour, and he has multiple haemorraghes surrounding the tumour. The pressure of the tumour has shifted the midline of his brain over to the right hand side (it needs to remain central to ensure he has full brain function) ... It doesn't matter what is done now, our little boy has already got permanent brain damage, and by the way the doctors were talking about it, it's SERIOUS permanent brain damage.

BUT that doesn't matter to us. Regardless of his condition we will love him endlessly. He is our little boy. He's our son. Nothing is going to change that. Nothing is going to change the love we have for Otis.

Things will change, yes. But as long as we have him here with us, we honestly couldn't care less. I would walk to the ends of the Earth on hot coal for this little boy growing within me. He already is my entire world, alongside the girls.

Speaking of which, I haven't seen the girls properly in weeks with all this going on. I feel like such a bad mummy right now. Not only am I neglecting Cora and Maisie by not seeing them, I have failed Otis. I have failed to grow him safely. I cannot help feeling like this is my fault. I probably always will. Watching him grow up with this damage to his poor self is going to break my heart; but he's already proven how strong-willed and stubborn he is. He has already proven how much of a fighter he is. I have no doubt in my mind he will continue fighting.

May 25th 2016.

Dear Diary,

We are going to lose our little boy.

We got called to an urgent meeting today with the neurologist and a doctor. On arrival, there just happened to be a bereavement midwife greet us. I knew, instantly, what they were going to tell us.

'I'm sorry. Your little boy has a serious tumour engulfing over ¾ of his brain. He also has multiple haemorraghes taking over his brain as well as a shift in the midline of his brain. Due to the severity of the haemorraghes, your little boy is not going to make it. He has no chance. I'm sorry.'

Our son, our precious Otis, is incompatible with life. He isn't going to live. He isn't even going to get the chance. He won't ever be able to breathe on his own. He won't be born alive.

June 1st 2016.

Dear Diary,

I'm back at the hospital.

My dad and Chris have just left for the night, ready for me to be induced tomorrow. Water has always been my calm. If ever I need to relax or need time to think, I'll have a bath or shower. The day has been stressful, so I'll jump in the shower to try and wind down. I need to sleep –

tomorrow is going to be a long, hard day. I doubt I'll be getting much sleep once he arrives, I mean, newborns rarely sleep, let's be honest!

I'm in the shower, just about to wash my hair and my water-loving little boy isn't moving. For the first time since he first started kicking and wriggling in my tummy, I'm not feeling him move in the shower. He loves water. Why isn't he moving? I poked and prodded, trying to get him to move for me. I feel one tear escape my eyes and roll down my cheek. *Come on, Otis. Just one little kick and I'll leave you alone. Stop being silly now.* He still isn't moving. Why isn't he moving? I can't usually have a shower in peace. This is the one time I want him to kick me and he won't. He must just be a stubborn monkey, like his big sister Cora. I prod my tummy again, trying to make him mad so he kicks my finger away like he was doing yesterday. He loves playing that game with me. He's so cheeky. Another tear rolls down my cheek … Maybe I should call the midwife in? Am I overreacting? Something doesn't feel right. Otis isn't moving – there must be something wrong with him. Why isn't he moving? *Come on, Otis. Come on. Move! Kick me. Just one little wriggle. Let me know you're okay. Please, little boy. Just one kick and I'll stop poking and prodding you, I promise.* He still isn't moving. I'm begging him. *Otis, please.*

Nothing.

I fall to my knees. I feel heaviness on my chest, like someone is pushing on it. I struggle breathing; it feels like I'm being suffocated. Then from somewhere deep, deep inside I muster up the strength to scream. I shout. *NO! NO! NO!* The tears are starting to properly flow now. The water from the shower is pouring over my face, tears that are pouring are stinging my eyes, my sopping wet hair is falling in front of my face. I try to reach up to grab the cord to call for a midwife. I feel like I'm going to die. I genuinely think this is it. This has to be the end. It hurts so bad. This pain in my chest; it's unbearable. I try to grab the cord but I can't see properly. I can't make anything out around me in that bathroom.

NO! Otis, NO! Please, God. No. Not my little boy. Please, please, don't take him with you. I NEED him. I NEED him more than you! Please, leave him here. Take me instead if you have to, just leave my little boy. PLEASE.

Nothing.

I fall from my knees on to my side. I curl into a ball and grab my tummy. I squeeze around my bump so, SO hard. *Otis, please move. Don't let it be true. Don't let the doctor be right. You haven't gone. Have you? Otis?*

I'm cuddling this perfect little boy in my tummy. *This can't be it, Otis. You were made out of love. You blessed our lives with your little life because you're going to do great things. You're going to grow up with your big sisters. You cannot leave us, Otis. You can't. Please. Don't go.*

It's too late, isn't it? He's really gone. They weren't lying to me this morning, were they? *You're really gone, aren't you, Otis? You're dead, aren't you?*

I can't find the strength to scream. I need to scream but it just won't come out. I try, so hard. The need to scream is overwhelming but all that escapes my mouth is a harsh whisper. *NO. No. No. Please, no. This can't be the end of you, Otis.*

I crawl out of the shower and sit, still completely naked, up against the wall of the bathroom. I don't feel capable to stand. I don't feel strong enough to support my own weight right now. I need to just sit here. I need to sit here and wait for this to be over.

But it's never going to end, is it? This is going to define me for the rest of my fucking life. People are going to look at me. People are going to know what's happened and they're going to look at me differently. I've changed. In the last few minutes of realising I'm now the mother to a child who will be born in to Heaven, I've changed. I will never be the same again. I know that already.

…

It feels like hours have passed and I'm still sat on this bathroom floor. I need to move. I get up and try to steady myself against the wall. My knees are shaking beneath me. I know I'm not going to physically be able to stay standing for long. I somehow find the strength to drag myself to the bed and collapse in a heap on to it.

I can't stop crying. Where are these tears even coming from, now? Surely I have no more left to cry.

June 2nd 2016

Dear Diary,

Okay, so my eyes are open. It's light outside. What time is it? 6am. Not that bad of a sleep, considering. I must have cried myself to sleep last night.

The midwife has just been in to say goodbye; her shift is ending in a couple of hours and she doesn't want to keep oining me, so says goodbye, wishes me luck and leaves me to it. I'm thankful. I need to sit in silence and enjoy the last few hours of having my little boy where he belongs – safe and warm inside my tummy. With me.

Chris and dad have arrived. They're both sat in the living area of the suite, I'm starting to feel a few niggling contractions, but nothing painful. I don't think this is it, just yet. The midwife has just knocked on the door. I'll be back.

...

Okay, so it's just after 11am and I've been induced. They give me gel just inside my cervix. They're hoping it'll soften and open my cervix gently over the next 24 hours. It already seems to be working though. Seriously, I'm contracting every 3 minutes already! They're getting more painful with each one. Can't say I'm excited about the rest of this labour, to be honest. For more reasons than the obvious agony I'm going to be dealing with.

Dad has just nipped home for a shower and some food. Chris is sat watching TV in the living area, helping himself to my biscuits with his brew. Shower time. Maybe that will help the pain a little. Worth a try I suppose.

Bad idea. He still isn't moving.

It seems this bathroom floor has become my new 'spot' ... This floor has seen me at my most honest. It's 'easier' to put on a brave face in front of dad and Chris. I can't keep crying – I need to stay strong for them. It isn't fair for them to see me constantly breaking down.

This floor, on the other hand, this floor doesn't give a shit. This floor can see whatever side of me I want it to see. This floor can see me being weak. This floor can see my soul. This floor can see the rawness of this reality. This floor can see every single tear. This floor can see me vulnerable. This floor can see my core. This floor can see the honesty of this situation.

Please don't let this be it. I'm your mummy. I'm supposed to look after you. It's my duty to protect you. It's my job as your mummy to get you here safe and sound and I haven't even managed to do that. I have failed you, Otis. I'm sorry. I'm really, really sorry. Please, forgive me.

Agony.

Please, God. PLEASE take me, instead. Take the air out of my own lungs and give it to my little boy! Take the blood out of my veins and put it in to his. Take the sight from my eyes and hand it to him. Take the taste out of my mouth and put it in his. PLEASE. I am BEGGING you! If you really exist, WHY are you doing this to me? Why are you doing this to us?! Why are you doing this to HIM!? WHAT has my poor, innocent, perfect little boy ever done? What harm has he caused to the world that he so deserves to DIE? If you really exist, take me. Take ME. Fucking take me!!!! Leave him alone. Just leave him. PLEASE.

I wonder how many people have led on this bathroom floor, crying in to their hands, begging for God to take them instead of their child? I wonder how many wounds of different women scar the walls of this bathroom? I wonder how many wounds of different men scar the floor of this bathroom? I wonder how many women have done the same as I do now – lying at their most vulnerable on this bathroom floor, completely naked, sopping wet through, cradling their pregnant tummy, hoping and praying to a God they aren't sure they even believe in, to work miracles and breathe life back in to their child?

This isn't fair. I can't do this. *Please, Otis. Wake up.*

Nothing.

June 4ᵗʰ 2016.

Dear Diary,

Yesterday our beautiful little boy, Otis Dominic Anthony Cullen graced the Earth. He is so perfectly beautiful. I have him led here, beside me, asleep. Asleep, as he will be forever.

Here's my birth story …

Otis was a fully formed, viable human being. I was over 35 weeks pregnant when his heart stopped beating. He wasn't just going to be absorbed back in to my body, or expel himself from my womb. I had to be induced, I had to go through labour, and I had to push that little boy out just like I would have if he was alive.

It was completely terrifying.

Childbirth is difficult enough in itself without the added terror of giving birth to your sleeping baby. Knowing that every single agonising contraction was leading to our first hello with our little boy was too hard to comprehend, then knowing that once we had met him we were going to be counting down to our last good bye; it was simply soul destroying..

Just a prior warning that from here on out, it's going to be pretty raw.

I was induced properly at 11am on the Thursday. They inserted a gel into my cervix in the hope that over the course of 24 hours it would gently soften my cervix and slowly induce labour. This didn't happen for me! Within seconds of having that gel inserted I started contracting, and I stared contracting thick and fast. Contractions were coming every 3 minutes from the word go, lasting over 1 minute each time. I grin and bared the pain for around 5 hours with no pain relief in the bereavement suite of the hospital – I was too scared to ask for pain relief because I knew if I had any that I'd have to be moved in to a normal delivery room, due to my medical history. Come 4(ish)pm, the pain was just getting too much. This wasn't necessarily in a physical way, but I couldn't hack it mentally. I remember saying to Chris that I wanted gas and air, because when I laboured with the twins it made my mind go elsewhere, and I didn't want to be where I was anymore. He called the midwife in for me and asked them if I could have the gas and air, they agreed because no pain relief is off limits when your child has no heartbeat.

They told me they'd return in a few minutes once they had prepped the delivery room next door. I kept thinking to myself 'what is there to prep? They're always ready' … On walking in the room, I understood. They had removed any equipment that would be used in a live delivery for the baby. They took out the rescusotation incubator, they removed suction equipment, they even took out the stethoscope … As thankful as I was that they were taken out of the room, it just made it that little more real that my baby wasn't going to be born alive.

Devastatingly, I still didn't even believe them at this point that he had died. I still insisted to myself that he was going to be born alive, that they had made a horrible mistake.

I started with the gas and air and it was great, it didn't ease the physical pain of the contractions at all, but it took my mind elsewhere which is what I needed. I sent Chris out at this point to get some food for him and my dad, who was waiting in the bereavement suite next door to us for Otis to arrive.

He returned about 30 minutes later, and after he had finished scoffing his kebab he came and sat in a chair next to me and grabbed my hand, where he remained for the rest of my labour, grabbed hand and all.

My mind was all over the place during this stage of my labour: one minute I was excited, forgetting that he was sleeping and the next minute I was terrified. There were so many conflicting emotions running through my mind and I was really starting to struggle with coping. I remember repeatedly shouting to the midwife that I simply couldn't do it. "I can't do it, I just can't."

I couldn't bare to see Otis sleeping, when he had been growing and living and kicking me just days before. When I had heard his heartbeat just days before..

Not much happened between then and 8pm, when the midwives did a shift swap. This is when I met Nicola, the woman who later delivered our baby. She was lovely. She became my rock throughout my labour and I genuinely don't think I would have got through it without her. I remember Nicola examining me around 8:30pm, but I can't remember how dilated I was. I was getting really sleepy at this point and asked for more pain relief. I was offered morphine.

Morphine?

"I didn't think you were allowed morphine during labour? Are you sure I'm allowed that?" … I was told yes. I was allowed anything I liked because no pain relief is off limit when your baby doesn't have a heartbeat. Initially, I turned it down. Admittedly, I know a massive part of me was punishing myself. I felt like I deserved the pain. I felt like I deserved to be in agony. I failed my son. I didn't grow him "right." I deserved to feel every last agonising second of every last contraction.

I broke down. Nicola comforted me and told me that none of this was my fault, that I didn't have to punish myself and didn't have to be uncomfortable. I looked at Chris, and he looked back at me as if to say "please, Nat, just have the morphine" … I knew at this point that he was struggling too. Not only was he waiting for his first son to arrive, sleeping, he was having to watch me go through labouring him too. I squeezed his hand the hardest I ever have as if to tell him "it's okay, we can do this", and I agreed to a have a morphine pump. It was administered around 10pm.

There was no letting up. It didn't matter how many times I pushed the button to activate the pump, nothing happened. The pain didn't ease, if anything it got worse. I looked at my arm and saw it was swollen to twice its size. The IV had tissued, the morphine wasn't even getting in to my system. It made me cry, I felt like someone else was punishing me now. I felt like they, too, thought I was worthy of feeling this horrible pain. I was reassured that it wasn't the case, and an anaesthetist came to fit a new cannula. I had 4 at this point, 2 in each arm.

I was examined. It was 11pm, and I was 9cm dilated.

Shit.

That meant I was close. No. I wasn't ready.

"Please, please can I have an epidural. I can't do this. I'm not ready to meet him yet."

They agreed. Otis didn't have a heartbeat, so I didn't have a timescale providing I was coping okay. I thought having an epidural would allow me to put off pushing once I was fully dilated. It definitely did.

The epidural was administered immediately, and I rested. I say rested – I spent the whole time until his birth repeatedly saying "no" to myself. Crying to Chris that I didn't want to do it anymore. Shouting at him whenever he so much as moved – "no! Please don't leave me! Please don't go anywhere" – he wasn't even leaving the room, just getting comfortable in the chair he had been sat in all day and evening.

I could feel pressure to push, an immense pressure, for over 4 hours and I forced myself to ignore it. I forced myself to feel that pain because it was the last time I could fool myself into believing my little boy was still living.

04:02am. "Natalie. We need you to push."

Fuck.

Chris came to sit beside me (he was led on a bed they had brought in for him for 30 minutes beforehand).

He grabbed my hand and looked at me. "You can do this."

This part was strangely peaceful. Because of the length of time Otis had been sat ready to be born, it was quite straight forward. He was right there. I pushed for 17 minutes – 6 pushes and he was born. He didn't cry. They were right. My son was dead.

Otis was born at 04:19am. He came in to the world just as the sun was rising outside, in to silence. There was no rushing around, there was no shouting from any midwives that he needed rescusotation, there was no doctors running in to save my boy .. WHY WERE THERE NO DOCTORS RUNNING IN TO SAVE HIM?! Did they not care!?

'No, Natalie. Your son is dead and he isn't coming back.' I had to keep reminding myself.

Chris squeezed my hand so hard, hid under the hood of his hoodie, scared to look. Nicola asked me if I wanted to see Otis. Of course, I said yes. I had waited 35 long weeks to see his beautiful face. To see if he looked like either of his big sisters or if he looked like his daddy. Nicola wrapped our lifeless, silent baby in a towel and placed him on my chest.

My heart exploded with love for this little being. He was perfect. My perfect piece of me. Chris' perfect piece of him.

Chris stood up and came to the side of the bed where he could see Otis' face. He broke down. For the first time on our whole journey, since finding out Otis was poorly, he broke down.

I knew from the second he was placed in to my arms that I'd never want to let him go, knowing every cuddle was leading to the last cuddle I'd ever give his physical body broke me. I looked over at Chris, who had gone to the other side of the room at this point in shock, and it was then that it hit me. Our little boy was dead. I had lost my son, Chris had lost his first son, his first child. He was never going to cry, he was never going to laugh, he was never going to return home, he was never going to play with his big sisters, he would never even meet his uncle Max or his cousins, he would never grow up.

I would give the world to turn back to yesterday. It was the single most painful experience of my life and I don't ever expect anything to come close to it. But I would do it again in a heart beat, without hesitation.

Otis Dominic Anthony Cullen; we miss you, we love you, we will do both eternally.

June 6th 2016

Dear Diary,

I'm back home now. Otis was collected yesterday by the funeral director from the hospital. I didn't have the strength to share about our days in the hospital, really, I still don't. But I need to write this down so I don't forget anything. I want to remember all of it.

"What, you actually get to see the baby?!"

Since Otis was born, I have had a few close friends ask me what actually happens after delivering a stillborn baby. I'm guessing a few acquaintances and strangers have wanted to know the answer to that question, too. It's one of those things; unless you have been through it yourselves, or walked alongside someone going through it, you just don't know. I know I didn't before it happened to me. Don't get me wrong, I knew what stillbirth was, but I definitely didn't know what happened after the baby had been delivered.

Our little boy made his entrance in to the world at 04:19am on June 3rd 2016. He weighed, and will forever weigh, 5lbs1oz. I know I keep repeating this – but it helps for the people who have only just started reading my blog and don't know this information. Due to me having an epidural at the end of my labour (9cm dilated), I lost the use of my legs. Because of this, I had to stay in the delivery room I had given birth in (as opposed to going back in to the bereavement suite) for a few hours, until the epidural wore off.

My dad, who was sitting in the bereavement suite waiting for Otis to be born, came in to the delivery room about 30 minutes after our little boy arrived. As soon as he walked in the room he started taking pictures. This is something I wouldn't have done myself, and something I will be genuinely, eternally grateful for. It's thanks to my dad that I now have over 200 pictures of Otis to look back on. The pictures aren't posed, so they're very raw, which makes them all that much more special to me.

After my dad had come in to the delivery room, Chris left to go and tell his mum and dad that our little boy had arrived, so I just spent time holding him, cuddling him, sharing him with my dad. It was a special couple of hours between my dad and I; between a father, his daughter and his grandson. Dad was there while Nicola (our midwife) weighed Otis and measured him. He was a lot bigger than we were expecting! I will treasure those hours for the rest of my life.

It was around 9am that I started to get feeling back in my legs and asked to be moved back to the bereavement suite, I didn't like being in that delivery room once I had started coming round properly, it just didn't feel 'right' … I should have been there with my crying baby, saying hello for the first time and looking forward to watching him grow. I should have been wondering whether he was going to be laid back like his daddy, stubborn like his mummy, intelligent like his big sister Cora, or witty and super funny like his big sister Maisie. I should have been talking to Chris about whose eyes he had – but we never got to see them. The midwife who came on the day shift must have understood how I felt without asking me, because her and my dad lifted me in to a wheelchair and took me through to the bereavement suite. They both got me comfortable in the double bed I had in there, and my dad left to get something to eat and to have a shower.

For a couple of hours I was on my own with my little boy. It was during this time that the bereavement midwife, Louise, helped me dress Otis in to his one and only baby grow he ever wore. I also used the time to let my two closest friends know that he had arrived, that he was absolutely perfect, and I sent them a picture. I made the most of having this special time with Otis because I knew it was soon going to end.

What a lot of people don't know is that, when you give birth to a stillborn baby, you have to register them lawfully. You have to register their birth and death on the same day to receive a 'stillbirth certificate.' You have to register them before you can legally take your baby out of the hospital or have them picked up by a funeral director. Cruel – I know. As Otis was born on the Friday we HAD to get him registered that day, or we wouldn't be able to get an appointment until the Monday, and we wanted to get the ball rolling in terms of organising a pick up day with the funeral directors we had chosen (Champs of Clayton–Le–Moors).

After Otis was born we had the choice as to whether we wanted to stay in the hospital with him, go home with him, or go home without him. I chose to stay at the hospital, where I felt it was safe to have him. I was scared of taking him home. I was worried about only being able to associate home with having my dead child there, and I didn't want that. It wouldn't have been fair for me or the girls.

I was absolutely terrified of leaving the hospital on Friday, leaving Otis behind in the hospital on his own, to go and register him at the registry office. Thankfully it was organised for the lady at the office to come in to the hospital and register him for us. A small gesture, but an appreciated one nonetheless. She came out at about 11am and we registered our little boy's birth and death – Otis Dominic Anthony Cullen was officially a person, a human being.

At around dinner time on Friday, we had a photographer in to take some pictures of Chris and I with our little boy. It was uncomfortable, it felt strange and a little forced, but I am SO thankful that Claire (our photographer) came to us to do it. Thanks to her we have some stunning pictures of us all together, and some of Otis on his own, that we can keep forever. These pictures that Claire took captured our emptiness but our undying love for Otis.

It was around 2pm that day that Maisie and Cora came to the hospital to meet their little brother, for the first and last time. Seeing them walk through that door with such excitement on their faces to meet him absolutely broke my heart. I don't think they understood at this point that their baby brother was never coming home. It was also at this time that my little sister Zoe came to meet her baby nephew, for the first and last time. She held him, she kissed him, she loved on him as she would have if he was alive. I would give anything for her and the girls to have had more time with him, I really would.

Chris' parents came to visit Otis that evening. It was emotional to say the least. My family were 'lucky' in a sense because they had been involved with my pregnancy from the get go. My sister had seen him at scans that Chris couldn't make it to, and had therefore seen him alive. Chris' parents hadn't had that opportunity for one reason or another – we didn't think it mattered that much, because as far as we knew, they'd spend all the time in the world with Otis when he was born. To this day, not involving them more in my pregnancy is one of my biggest regrets. Hindsight is a beautiful thing, isn't it? They held Otis, they cried, they hugged, they apologised (for what I don't know). Otis would have been their first grandson – their first grandchild. They were beyond devastated. I cannot put in to words the love I saw they had for Otis just by being in that room with them when they met him. It's a sight I will never, ever forget.

After Chris' parents left, my step mum Sam came to visit. It was hard to see her cry because I've never seen her cry before. She gave Otis big cuddles and repeatedly told me that it isn't fair.

This was probably something I needed to hear at that point, because it wasn't. It really wasn't fair. At all. Sam's visit with Otis was short, but sweet. She was hesitant about coming to see him at first, and I'm very glad that she did. I think if she had decided not to, that it would be a big regret later down the line. As dad told me 'you can always forget a memory you don't want to remember, you cannot make up memories that never happened.' In other words, if Sam wanted to ever 'forget' meeting Otis then she could, she could never have turned back the clock and changed her mind to meet him if she hadn't met him that day. Wow, I'm babbling.

After Sam left my big sister Jayde came to visit. She had her cuddles and kisses, and said hello and goodbye to Otis. Jayde and I had only just started rekindling our relationship properly the few months before Otis was born, and I'm happy that she came to meet and love on mine and Chris' little boy.

Everybody left and it was just Chris and I left with Otis. I knew that he was struggling to be around him much, it's hard for anyone to see their child after they have passed away. I think Chris found it difficult knowing that there was nothing he could do to help his little boy. Otis is his first son; his first child. Men tend to see it as their 'duty' to protect their children, and Chris was powerless to help Otis. There was absolutely nothing he could have done to save him – I think, knowing him like I do, that this made him feel weak, and helpless, and being around Otis too much reminded him of that. He did push past that and made the most of the time we had with our little boy at the hospital.

At around 1am Chris left the hospital and I was, again, left alone with Otis.

It was strange. Although he had passed away I felt content having him in my arms. I felt content that I could pick him up and cuddle him, kiss him and love him whenever I pleased. I didn't cry much that night. This was partly due to the shock and partly due to the fact I had no tears left to cry.

On Saturday, Chris, my dad and my friend Mel came up to the hospital. Mel was the only one of my friends who came to see Otis and I will be forever thankful that she did. She was the only one of my friends who had the guts to face me. The only one of my friends that had the strength to come and hold my little boy. It meant the world to me and it always will. Mel spent a couple of special hours crying with me, holding Otis, speaking to him, loving him and loving me. The Saturday was pretty calm. We had Otis' footprints and handprints done, a cast made of his hand and foot, and plenty more pictures were taken. I then just spent the day cuddling him, while Chris waited on me hand and foot making sure I was fed and watered, making sure I was comfortable etc. After dad and Mel left it was just Chris and I alone with our little boy and our thoughts. We had a good heart to heart that night, about how proud we were (and still are) of our little boy for making it as far as he did despite the odds being stacked against him. We spoke about regrets we had from during the pregnancy (me complaining I was tired, him missing a couple of scans due to work – which in hindsight was just not that important, if we knew earlier that those scans were the only time we would see our son alive, then work would have taken a back seat, 100%).

Chris stayed with Otis and me until around 11pm that evening. He decided against staying in the hospital with me, despite being given the choice, to let me spend quality time with Otis on my own. I thank him for that, because it was during those night time hours that I led and cried in to my babies chest. It was during those night time hours that I led cuddling Otis and sang him lullabies; the same ones that I used to sing to the girls when they were babies. It was during those hours that I apologised to Otis over and over for failing his beautiful little self. It was during those night time hours that I held him to my chest, my bare skin, like I would had he been born alive. It was during those night time hours that I bonded with my son.

We were given the choice on the Saturday as to whether we wanted to leave the hospital before Otis, at the same time as Otis, or after Otis. We decided to leave at the same time as him for two reasons:
 1.) So he didn't get taken down to the morgue to be left there until he was collected.
 2.) So he wasn't being taken out of the hospital without me. He wouldn't have left without me if he was alive, I refused to let it happen in death.

Morning came. *I sit in tears as I write this.* Morning came, and it was the day that Otis was being picked up by the funeral director. It was the day I had to cuddle my son for the very last time.

I spent the Sunday morning loving Otis, wiping his little face with some warm water on soft tissue, cutting off his cord clamp to keep as I did with the girls, taking off one of his hospital bands to put in my memory box, and changing him in to his burial outfit.

I was told that the funeral director or a midwife would do it for me, but I insisted. It was one of the very few things I could do for my little boy and I WAS going to do it. I spoke to him as I changed him from his baby grow in to a beautiful little burial gown, waistcoat and all. He looked stunning. But it broke my heart. My little boy's second ever outfit, and last outfit, was his burial outfit.

12:30 midday came. It was time.

I picture now, the funeral director walking in to my bedroom with that moses basket in tow. How was this fair?! The one and only time I would place my little boy in to a moses basket and it was to take him to a funeral home. It took every ounce of strength I had not to collapse in a heap on the floor. I held Otis tight to my chest, gave him a kiss and told him that I loved him before placing his tiny body into the moses basket. How I had the capability to stay standing at that point is beyond me. I broke down in to my dads chest. We looked at our little boy laying in that moses basket for a few minutes, I took in every last millimetre of his beautiful little face.

Then it happened ...

My dad asked Chris if he wanted to carry Otis to the funeral car waiting outside, he couldn't – I don't think he felt he had the strength. So my dad did it. He picked up Otis in the little moses basket and carried him out of the delivery suite, down the corridor to the lift, out of the lift, down the corridor to the back entrance of the hospital, to the funeral car waiting outside. He carried his little grandson for the very last time.

I'm going to the funeral home this afternoon, to plan our son's funeral, and to see him for the very last time. I'll speak later.

June 6th 2016.

Dear diary,

It's only been a few hours since I last wrote. A LOT has happened in the last few hours. They've been the most harrowing of my entire life.

'In my professional opinion, I wouldn't recommend that anybody come see Otis now.' – The words spoken by our funeral director just three days after our little boy was born, just after I'd finished writing my last entry a few hours ago.

It was Lianna (our funeral director) telling my dad that she didn't want anyone going down to see Otis, as he had deteriorated too much, too quickly.

This is, in part, due to the fact that the cuddle cot at the hospital that was supposed to keep Otis' body refrigerated enough to 'preserve' him, was not turned on the whole time we were there. I was, obviously, completely oblivious. I thought that it would have been on, I had never been around a dead baby before so I guessed that it was normal for Otis to deteriorate and change as much as he did in just two days. Apparently not.

My heart shattered hearing those words.

I left hospital with Otis just yesterday, assuming that I would be able to spend time with him during this week at the funeral home. Because of this, I didn't say a 'proper' goodbye to him at the hospital, so I went against Lianna's recommendation and insisted I see my little boy today, one last time.

We had arranged to go down at 2pm today to sort out Otis' funeral anyway, and it had also become the time that I would be seeing Otis for the first time in the funeral home, and the last. After deciding what we wanted for the funeral, Lianna took us through to see Otis. She asked me *'are you sure you want to do this?'* … Of course, I said yes. I didn't care what he looked like, I HAD to see him to say goodbye properly.

My dad, Chris and I walked in to the room and saw his little moses basket. I was terrified to walk over but I found strength somewhere within me and forced myself to go and stand next to him. Chris struggled to see his little boy in there, and sat in the corner of the room on a chair. I looked down in to the moses basket. He looked perfect. He looked so perfectly peaceful and beautiful. He was cuddling his little teddy Chris had bought me for Mother's Day when I was pregnant; he had his little wolly hat on and was wrapped in a nice thick blanket, to keep him warm.

But he was blue. Upon leaving the hospital just yesterday, Otis still had a lot of pink skin, as well as the blue tinge. By this afternoon he had turned completely blue and because of the way nature works, he had also started to let off a pungent smell.

It was devastating.

As horrible as it is to say this; just a couple of hours ago I was looking at my little boy decomposing in front of my eyes.

It broke me. I broke down. I just wanted to reach in to the moses basket and pick him up, hold him tight to my chest and stay there forever, protecting him. I wanted to change the course of nature and stop this happening to my little boy; but I couldn't even pick him up – he was too fragile. I cried in to my dad's chest, then as I pulled away, hands shaking, I took the ring off my finger that Chris had bought me three years ago and placed it around two of Otis' tiny fingers – his middle finger and ring finger … Then I put Chris' bracelet that I bought him three years ago in Otis' other hand. I placed the letters that Chris and I wrote him at the bottom of the moses basket and the teddies off the girls beside his head. I asked for time alone with him, and my dad and Chris left the room.

The second they walked out of that room I collapsed in a heap on the floor next to the moses basket. I didn't have the strength in me to stay strong anymore. I wanted to take his place. I cried as I knelt beside the moses basket, holding Otis' hand. I pleaded for this not to be the last time I would ever see him. I begged and begged for it to be me taking his place and nothing happened. I prayed so hard (if there really is a God) for him to breathe my life in to Otis; to take the air out of my lungs and put it in to my little boys lungs. I had already had a chance at living; I honestly did not care. I would have given ANYTHING to take his place and it be me lying in that funeral home, I still would! But nothing happened. This was my reality. It really was my little boy who was being taken away.

I whispered in to his ear:

'I'm so sorry that I failed you. This shouldn't be happening. Please, don't be scared baby. You're going to be okay. Your grandmas, granny and grandad will look after you when you get to where you're going. There's no need to be scared. I love you, we love you.'

I stroked his little head and quietly sang (through a lot of tears) the little lullaby I sang to the girls when they were babies, and still sing to them now when they're poorly, before saying to him: *'goodnight baby, sleep well and sweet dreams.'*

I planted a gentle kiss on his forehead. I planted a gentle kiss on his cheek. Then I planted a gentle kiss on his lips. I stroked his tiny ear and touched his little fingers one last time… Then I walked out of the room without turning back to look at him. I knew if I looked at him again that I would never be able to walk away.

Today has been the single, most harrowing day of my entire life so far. Giving birth to Otis broke me. Planning his funeral destroyed me. But saying goodbye to my precious boy's physical body, knowing that it would be the very last time I ever saw him is a pain beyond comprehension. I cannot begin to put in to words how it felt walking out of that room, away from him.

It went against every motherly instinct I had, walking away from my baby.

I hope he knows, wherever he is, how difficult it was for me to do that. I hope he knows that I didn't want that day to be the last time I saw him, but I couldn't bare to see his perfect body decompose anymore in front of my eyes. I hope he knows that I would have spent every waking minute with him for the rest of my life if I could. I hope he knows that we miss him, that we love him and that we will do so eternally.

Otis' funeral has been planned for this Friday (the 10th). It's sudden, I know, but I just want it over and done with. I don't like the idea of my precious boy laying in that moses basket just a couple of roads away from me, knowing I can't go down to pik him up to cuddle and kiss him as I please.

June 8th 2016.

Dear Diary,

I didn't really speak much about planning Otis' funeral on Monday. There wasn't too many decisions to make; luckily my dad had taken care of the basics.

So here goes … *Planning our little boy's funeral* – wow, that is something I never thought I'd write. But no one does, do they? Losing a child was always my irrational fear, I remember always thinking *'it will never happen to me, it just doesn't happen to people like me'* … and it did. My most irrational fear is now my most rational, because it's my reality. It DID happen to me, and after it happened to me, I had to plan my son's funeral.

Otis was born last Friday morning, we spent two AMAZING days with our little boy before he was collected by the funeral directors on Sunday at midday. We chose to organise his funeral with Champs Funeral Services in Clayton-Le-Moors, and they are honestly nothing short of wonderful. The service they provide and compassion they show is second to none. I truly believe they will help make Otis' funeral on Friday as perfect as can be.

We decided to have Otis buried. I've come to learn that most parents of stillborn babies decide to have their child cremated. Having Otis buried is a decision I pushed on to Chris because I desperately want Otis to have his own little resting place – somewhere that I can go to recollect and speak to him, somewhere to be alone with my own thoughts, somewhere where his big sisters can go and play, somewhere people can visit without having to ask us first. Despite being a decision made in the midst of confusion, I know it's one I will not regret.

If Otis had lived we would have opted to have him Christened, just as his big sisters were Christened when they were babies. Because of this, it only felt 'right' that his funeral service be held in a church, as opposed to a crematorium, at his graveside or at the funeral home itself. Otis' service will take place at All Saints Church in Clayton-Le-Moors, the same Church his big sisters were Christened in. We have chosen for Otis to rest in a tiny blue coffin, decorated with animal stickers. His nursery is jungle themed, so it only felt 'right' that we carry this theme through to his forever bed.

Chris will carry Otis' coffin in to the church to Eva Cassidy's version of 'Over the Rainbow'. I am dreading seeing him holding Otis in his coffin, knowing it will be the very last time he will ever hold our son in his arms. I already know that watching Chris carry our little boy in to that church is going to be something I will never forget and it will be nothing short of agonising.

I wrote a letter to our little boy that will be read out during the service by the vicar as I don't have the strength to read it myself. We have also decided that his big sisters will light a candle for him during our time of recollection.

We have decided that Otis will be buried in a little 'baby garden' in a local cemetery. I have the ideology that with him being buried alongside other babies, he will never be alone. One of mine and his daddy's favourite songs (Otis Redding – Dock of the Bay) will be played at his graveside as his coffin is being lowered, and once his coffin is in the ground we will sprinkle glitter and stars on his coffin, as opposed to the usual 'ashes and dust'.

One of the hardest decisions during planning Otis' funeral was the songs we were going to use. It was difficult for two reasons:
 1.) Will the song be 'suitable'?
2.) How much do I like this song? Because I will never listen to it the same again.

And I can't. I cannot listen to Otis' funeral songs without breaking down already and it hasn't even happened yet. I can't listen to them without imagining his tiny, lifeless, beautiful body lying in that coffin. I can't listen to them without thinking about what we are missing out on; without thinking about who and what he would have become; without thinking about the fact I should now have a precious one month old baby in my arms.

Planning Otis' funeral was soul destroying, but it was the only one thing we would ever be able to do for our son as his parents. We won't ever be able to plan a birthday party, we won't ever be able to help him with his homework, his daddy won't ever be able to teach him how to ride a bike or how to fish (though he'd struggle with that because he can't really fish himself!).

The funeral is on Friday and I'm hoping and praying it goes by without a hitch and I really hope we have done Otis proud in organising his 'special' day for him.

Otis Dominic Anthony Cullen; we miss you, we love you & we will do both eternally.

June 10th 2016.

Dear Diary,

Just need to write a little something to my little boy after his precious service today. Everything went swimmingly. It was beyond heartbreaking. I don't have the words to come close to explaining how I feel right now; though I'm sure I will at a later date.

Otis Dominic Anthony Cullen ... Me and daddy hope we did you proud today. And we want you to know that today does not mark the end of your little story, we will speak of you for the rest of our lives - just because you aren't here with us doesn't mean you aren't important. You're our little boy, our beautiful son, and we will forever be grateful for the short time we had with you while you were in my tummy. Maisie and Cora will grow up to know their little brother, they'd have made you so proud with how strong they were today.

Your little face will forever be imprinted in my mind & we are happy we got to share it on a picture with everyone who attended today. Mummy, daddy, Cora and Maisie love you beyond words. Grandma Sue, Grandma Lilian, Granny and Grandad will look after you & tell you bedtime stories until we meet again. Rest well sweet boy.

We miss you, we love you, we will do both eternally.

June 15th 2016.

Dear diary,

I have a lot I need to say to my little boy today. I hope you don't mind.

Otis,

I cannot put in to words how much I miss you, sweet boy. There are no words in existence to describe how much I wish you were here with me, daddy and your big sisters.

You didn't deserve for this to happen to you. There are so many bad people in the world that have the chance to live and they take that for granted; and then someone as sweet, as innocent, as perfect and pure as you gets taken away. You did not deserve to leave the world before you got the chance to open your eyes and see it. You did not deserve for your tiny brain to be engulfed by a nasty tumour. You did not deserve for your perfect little body to be plagued by multiple haemorrhages. You did not deserve to only know your daddy and big sisters through hearing their voices. You did not deserve to die.

I would give my very last breath if it meant seeing you take just one, I really would. I know that your daddy would too. Yes, we are still young, but we have had a chance at life – you didn't even get that. Finding out that we were going to lose you tore my heart in half and I just haven't been the same since.

It doesn't feel 'right' existing without you. And I'm doing just that – *existing*. I'm not living, I'm barely coping without you here. I'm existing because I have to. I have a duty to look after your sisters, I have a duty to carry on being a mum and it's difficult. It scares me how difficult it has become. Not because I'm not capable – but because I am terrified of losing Cora or Maisie now, too. Having to bury one of my children was once just an irrational fear, but it's now my reality. It's completely rational because it has happened to me with losing you. I worry the second they leave my sight that it'll be the last time I ever see them alive. No mummy deserves this. No child deserves this.

I'm sorry that you had to go, I will feel forever guilty for not being able to grow you properly. I will always blame myself, regardless of how many people tell me to think otherwise. I feel like I have failed you. The first thing I was supposed to do as your mummy was make sure you arrived Earth side safe and sound, and healthy. I couldn't even do that. I'm not saying for a second that I didn't deserve to be given the chance, because I loved you from day dot. From seeing those two pink lines on that pregnancy test, you were my son. I DID deserve you, I DID deserve the chance to be your mummy.

All the way through my pregnancy with you I was fussy. I took for granted that you were living. I assumed that you were going to be born alive and because of that I never focused on just getting you here living. I focused on what I was going to do once you had been born – I was adamant that I would breastfeed, for example; I was adamant that you wouldn't be leaving my side over night for at least the first six months; I was adamant that you be born naturally instead of having a repeat caesarean. I would have had a caesarean and handed you to someone else overnight the day you were born if it meant having you with me. Those things just really did NOT matter. The things I thought most important in raising you just did NOT matter. What mattered is that you, a little person, a perfect human being, was safe and loved. What mattered is that you should have lived. I focused on your future instead of the 'here and now.' I wish I had just taken the time to focus on you as an unborn child, because that's the only time I ever had you alive. That's the only time you had a beating heart.

It doesn't feel 'right' not having you here in my arms. They ache to hold you. That's not metaphorical. I literally ache to feel your 5lbs1oz weight in my arms. It hurts, Otis. It really, really hurts. Mummy would do anything just to turn back to the day I first laid eyes on your beautiful but lifeless body, just to give you one more cuddle.

It doesn't feel 'right' not watching your big sisters love on you. They miss you so much. They speak of you every single day. The girls constantly look at your pictures and cuddle them; they ask about you and they wonder where you are – I do try my best to answer the questions they ask about you, it just gets hard sometimes. When I tell the girls I don't want to talk about it, it's not because I don't want to talk about YOU, I just cannot handle speaking your name sometimes. It hurts, Otis. But the love I have for you makes the pain worth it. I hope you know that.

The second I laid eyes on you my heart just exploded with love for you. I loved you already, but seeing you for the first time just took that love to another level. It would have been my instinct as your mummy to protect you for the rest of your life had you lived; I knew there and then, the minute you were born, that it would become my duty to protect your memory for the rest of MY life. And that, I will do. It is the least you deserve.

There are no words to describe how proud I am, as your mummy, that you didn't give up. You have the same fighting spirit that your big sisters do. That's one thing I do know about your personality. You fought so hard. I cannot begin to tell you how proud we all are of you for holding on, for fighting to meet us. I cannot begin to tell you how thankful I am that you didn't give up and you let me cuddle you, kiss you, hold you, say hello to you face to face.

I am happy that you passed away peacefully; I'm thankful that our bodies came together, entwined as one, to ensure that you passed away not in pain. I'm glad that you never knew fear and that you never will know fear. The world is a scary place, you will never have to experience that. All you ever knew was warmth and love.

We didn't choose for this to happen. When we found out I was pregnant with you, we didn't choose to become the parents and siblings of a little angel baby. We didn't choose to say hello and goodbye to you all in the same day. We didn't choose for your grandparents to lose their grandson, or your aunts and uncles to lose their nephew. We didn't choose for any of this. But if I had to do this all over again, if choosing and losing you meant having the chance to LOVE you, then I would pick for you to be our son again in a heart beat. I am BLESSED to be your mummy, I am thankful that we are your family, I am beyond honoured to have carried you within me.

I miss you, I love you, I will do both eternally.

Lots of love,

Mummy x

June 18th 2016.

Dear diary,

I'm feeling angry today. For many reasons I'm sure. Yesterday was Chris' birthday, and tomorrow is Father's Day. His first birthday as a daddy, his first Father's Day as a daddy, and the nearest he gets to spending those days with his son is sitting by his graveside. HOW is this fair?!

Today, a lady on a support group I'm a part of sent me a message. (Please note, I have been given permission to use her words). She said; *'please help me. I'm going crazy! I don't think the way I'm feeling is normal.'*

I asked her why; I asked her to be honest with me about how she felt. She proceeded to say; *'It's been 7 months since my little girl was born and I still cry every single day. I get angry at every one around me for absolutely no reason and when people ask me how I'm doing I really don't know how to answer because I don't know how I'm doing. Am I going mad? I can't even think straight anymore.'*

The most heart breaking part about receiving this message was knowing every single thought she has, every feeling that she feels; it is all completely normal. Rational? Maybe not to someone who has never given birth to their dead child. But, sadly, completely normal to those who have. Completely relatable to those who have …

I HAD to write after reading that message. It genuinely took some considerable time before it was definitive that I would share our story. Writing about Otis, especially so soon after losing him, is emotionally exhausting. It really does take it out of me; but after reading how this poor woman felt so isolated in how she feels I knew I had to do this. I had to write because I realised that there would be hundreds, if not thousands, of other women and men feeling the same way that she does, and I felt it my duty to reassure those people that there are so many variations of 'normal' when it comes to grieving for your child.

Losing a baby – giving birth to a fully formed, viable baby – then having to plan that baby's funeral, having to bury or cremate your child, is not within the 'normal' realms of the natural cycle of life. It should not happen. Biologically, we have it wired in to us that we will lose those close to us who are older than us. It's like we don't have a biological instinct on how to grieve for our babies. I know, from personal experience, that grieving after losing an older relative tends to be fairly 'straight-forward', if you will. It's hard, it's upsetting, we cry, it's painful to say goodbye, it's difficult to watch their coffin be lowered in to the ground; but it's something that you eventually move on from. Eventually.

It doesn't matter how many minutes, hours, days, weeks, months or years have passed, you just never move on from losing a child, you really don't. And for those who don't know this pain, do you want to know something? Believe it or not, that is completely 'normal.'

Every single time I feel a new emotion when it comes to my grieving for Otis, I reassure myself that it's okay to feel that way. Today, I feel a lot of anger, and that's fine! I feel like this after receiving a comment telling me that I speak of Otis like I'm the only person who has ever gone through stillbirth. This angered me for two reasons:
 1.) I do not do this just for myself; those around me know how determined I am to help people through my writing; about how I hope that my sharing of Otis' story not only provides comfort to those who are suffering the same loss, but that it educates the people around them on how to spare their feelings, and about the harsh reality of stillbirth.
 2.) It is fucking HARD to write this book. Forcing myself to remember every last detail of our experience is mentally exhausting, and I wouldn't be doing this just to make the world feel sorry for me. I force myself to remember to HELP others suffering, to SHOW those who may feel they're struggling with their emotions that how they feel is okay. To show people dealing with stillbirth that they are NOT alone.

You see, the world of a grieving parent is such an isolating one. You can be surrounded by all the family and friends in the world; you can see someone every minute of your waking day; you can go to playgroups and meet up with mum friends with your other children; you can bump in to someone at the shop and say hello; you can see a counsellor and talk about how you feel in depth; you can be cuddled every day by your family for reassurance; but you will STILL feel alone. And do you know something? That is completely 'normal' too.

This journey of grief is so confusing – it really would help if 'Becoming the Mother or Father of a Stillborn Baby' was an existing instruction manual. It really would help if we were 'taught' how to grieve. But we can't be. Every single person's journey of grief is so different. I have a friend, who gave birth to her daughter sleeping at 35 weeks gestation (the same as me with Otis), 3 months prior to me losing my little boy. She's probably the closest I have to the circumstances surrounding Otis' death and you'd therefore think that we are grieving similarly.

If you do think that, you think wrong. Despite being completely relatable; despite knowing the EXACT pain one another is feeling; we are dealing with the death of our children completely differently. I'm putting the time I would have spent being a mummy to Otis in to writing, doing charity work and trying my God damn hardest to raise awareness on this awful, awful experience. My friend spends most of her days inside, crying in to the chest of her little girl's teddy bear that stores her ashes. And do you know something? THAT, is also completely 'normal.'

I've been told countless times that I'm 'strong' because I'm not spending all my days cooped up crying over the loss of my son. I've been told over and over again how I'm amazing because I'm dealing with Otis' death in an admirable way. For those who think that – I cry myself to sleep every night; I cannot visit my son's grave without my sister, my brother-in-law, Chris or my dad; I cannot look at another baby without crying for my own; I cannot go to the shop for fear of bumping in to someone I know … Putting on a brave face does not make me a strong person – it's my coping mechanism. Just like my friend's coping mechanism is to cry all day, most days. To COPE is all that matters, regardless of how it's achieved. She is strong, too.

I literally beg inside most days for this stage of my grief to pass – to skip to the part where I find my new normal and learn to live with Otis' passing away. It makes me feel guilty (again, another completely 'normal' emotion to feel). I know I only feel that way because of how agonising the pain is while it's so raw. I know I only feel that way because I don't WANT to feel this dagger through my heart every single morning when I wake up and realise it wasn't a dream; that my son is dead. I didn't CHOOSE for this to happen. It's okay for me to not want to feel this pain.

But then, I invite it. This pain makes me feel close to Otis. This raw, physical ache makes me really FEEL that I miss him. I invite the grief, I invite the crying, I invite the emptiness, I invite the sadness. The longing I have to hold my son; that's the one thing that makes me realise I'm still his mummy, regardless of where he is now. The pain in my chest and the aching of my arms to hold my son; it reassures me that he was HERE. That he DID exist. That he was (and is) a little person who DID grace the Earth, even if he didn't stay too long.

I have grown so much over the last 42 days since Otis was born sleeping. I see the world so differently now; I see life in general so differently. I have ALWAYS appreciated Cora and Maisie (my two girls) and I know how lucky I am to have these beautiful children in my life, but my appreciation for their existence has increased ten-fold. I cannot even look at them without counting my blessings.

When I got told Otis was going to die its like a switch flipped in my head and I changed. I actually could probably tell you to the second when I realised I'd never be the same again.

I guess what I'm trying to say is:
 For those who live every single day with an unbearable amount of conflicting feelings; know that it's normal, that it's okay and that you aren't alone.
 For those who have never been unfortunate enough to deal with this pain; be kind. Be kind to those you know who do. Realise that, such an event will probably have changed your friend, sister, brother, child etc. Understand that they won't be the same person they were before their child's heart stopped beating; understand even more that they will probably NEVER go back to being that person, so don't try to make them.

Otis Dominic Anthony Cullen; we miss you, we love you, we will do both eternally.

June 22nd 2016.

Dear Diary,

I'm writing this entry today in the hope that Chris reads it. I know he feels a lot of guilt for what's happened to our little boy. I know he feels he may have failed as a father by not being able to protect him. I feel like a letter off Otis is the only thing that may offer him some reassurance...

Dear Daddy,

I know that saying *'goodbye'* to me – your first son, your first child, before having the chance to say *'hello'* has caused you unimaginable pain. I know that losing me has been hard. I know that, as my daddy, you see it as your duty to protect me and to make sure that I'm okay. I know that me not being down on Earth with you and mummy hurts you badly. I know that not being able to help me makes you feel weak and helpless.

I want you to know that I'm being looked after by mummy's Grandmas, Sue and Lilian, as well as Granny and Grandad Cullen; I have made friends here too with the little girls and boys gone before me. Here, my eyes are open and I can see! Heaven is such a beautiful place. I'm not scared, daddy. I'm looking down on you and mummy from afar, and I know that one day I will see you again.

One day, you will see me with my eyes open, daddy. One day you will see me move. One day you will hear my cry. One day you will hear my laugh that you so long to hear.

I'm proud to call you my daddy. I often point you out to all the other angel babies and tell them who you are … *'Look! There's my daddy. He's so brave. He's so strong.'*

Thank you for not fighting me daddy. Thank you for not insisting the doctors deliver me the day you found out I was poorly, knowing that there was over 99% chance I would pass away immediately. Thank you for being completely unselfish and not insisting I was born that day, just for the 0.01% chance that I would have lived for few seconds and then die in front of yours and mummy's eyes, in pain. Thank you for allowing nature to take it's course and for letting me go gently in mummy's tummy, where all I knew was love and warmth. Thank you for making mummy see that this is the way it had to be.

I understand why you and mummy made that decision, daddy. I understand that you didn't want to see me suffer and waiting for my heart to stop beating inside mummy's tummy was the most loving act the both of you could have done. I understand that you knew I wouldn't have lived longer than a few seconds; if I even made it through the birth. I know that you knew those few seconds would have been absolutely agonising for me, and you let me go where I was pain free. You let me go where I had never known fear. I will always thank you for that.

I know that watching mummy go through all that immense pain, and watching me come in to the world silent was like a dagger through your heart. I know up to that point that a part of you still believed the doctors were wrong and I would be born with air in my lungs and crying. I know that the silence in the room when I arrived Earth side was devastating for you. I'm so proud of you, daddy, for staying so strong – even if you don't feel like you did at the time.

Thank you for looking after my mummy. Thank you for being there when she has needed a shoulder to cry on. Thank you for being there when I came in to the world with my eyes closed. Thank you for holding mummy's hand when she needed your guidance and your support. Thank you for standing by mummy's side when my little coffin was being lowered in to the ground.

Thank you, daddy, for facing your biggest fear and carrying me home.

Thank you for finding the strength you have always carried inside you and carrying me in my coffin in to the church when you didn't feel you could. I know it meant a lot to you that you held me one last time.

I know that you now miss out on the rest of your life with me. You were looking forward to watching me grow; teaching me how to ride a bike; teaching me how to play football; taking me to my first concert and on my first 'boys' holiday. You were excited to get to know the gentleman that you and mummy would have raised me to be. You were apprehensive, you were nervous, you were wondering how you would do it, but you love me. You love me, daddy, and that's all that mattered.

Mummy always talked to me when I was in her tummy, and she would often tell me how she was so excited to watch you become a daddy for the first time. She knew you were going to be an amazing one. You are an amazing daddy. You may not be able to hold me, you may not be able to sit up all night with me crying trying to console me, you may not be able to comfort me when I'm sick or after a nasty doctor gives me injections, you may not be able to cuddle me when I need you or kiss my knees better when I fall down, you may not be able to do the things that people assume good daddies do. But you love me. You help keep my memory alive, you honour the fact that I existed, you speak of me daily and come to see me at my resting place all the time. You didn't only love me in life, you love me in death. That, daddy, makes you amazing. Daddies to angel babies can be the best daddies, too.

Daddy, please know that I'm doing okay, and that there was nothing at all you could have done to save me. I know that, if yours and mummy's love alone could have saved me, I would have lived forever.

I look forward to the day that I see you again and I can teach YOU how to jump on the clouds and soar upon rainbows!

I love you daddy.

Your little boy, your little miracle,
 Otis x

June 25th 2016.

Dear Diary,

I'm feeling quite upset today.

"You are lucky. You knew he was going to die so you had time to prepare."

Shockingly, yes, those words have been said to me (and I quoted, word for word). I felt the need to share something after reading those words.

We had Otis' burial outfit delivered on the 28th of May, 2016 after confirming we wanted it on the 26th of May, 2016. Otis wasn't born until the 3rd of June, 2016. Receiving this outfit was by far one of the most harrowing experiences of my life … Opening that package and seeing the tiny outfit that I knew my little boy was going to rest in for the whole of eternity broke me in to a million pieces. Knowing that this little boy was still living and kicking inside me, knowing that he still had a heart beat, and I was sat looking at this beautiful gown in front of me that would become his burial outfit, was a feeling of pain beyond comprehension.

I cannot begin to explain that pain, I really can't.

Let me tell you.. There is NOTHING lucky about losing a child or knowing you're going to lose a child. There is NOTHING lucky about getting to 34 weeks of pregnancy to then hear; "I'm sorry, your son isn't going to live." There is NOTHING lucky about finding a funeral director before your

son has even passed away to make things as cope able as possible after birth. There is NOTHING lucky about waiting for your little boys heart to stop beating, knowing it's inevitable. There is NOTHING lucky about spending every second of every minute of every hour of every day waiting for the next kick, just to know he was still alive. There is NOTHING lucky about receiving a memory box for your child before they have even become a memory. There is NOTHING lucky about feeling your son kick, then realising later that it was for the very last time. There is NOTHING lucky about hearing those words; *'I'm sorry, there's no heartbeat. I'm so sorry for your loss.'* There is NOTHING lucky about my child dying – regardless of HOW or WHY or WHEN.

Yes, we had time to prepare for our sons heart to stop beating. This did NOT make our experience any easier! Getting to 34 weeks of pregnancy thinking that everything was okay, thinking that in just a few short weeks we would be bringing home our little boy to meet his sisters, thinking about who he would become, having a caesarean date planned to deliver my son ALIVE and HEALTHY … to THEN learn our darling boy would never be coming home – that is NOT lucky. Knowing I would have to deliver his lifeless body and having to prepare for that; even going to the lengths of researching how cold and floppy he would be when he arrived earth side – that is NOT lucky.

I cannot explain this feeling to those who have never experienced it. But now, after reading those words written to me, I'm gonna damn well try.

If you're a mummy or a daddy, imagine this:
 Imagine that little boy or girl you call your son or daughter. Imagine never having seen their eyes. Look at their eyes, and imagine having never seen those perfect eyes open. Now picture your beautiful son or daughter playing and think about their little laugh; imagine having never heard that laugh. You're led down in bed at night and you hear your child cry; imagine never having heard that cry. Do you remember the first time your little boy or girl said *'mama'* or *'dada'* ? Now imagine never hearing them say those words. You're lying in bed at night, cuddling your sleepy baby – now imagine holding that perfect piece of you tight to your chest, almost suffocatingly, and giving them a kiss goodbye knowing that it would be the very last time you do. You're putting your little one to bed, you stroke their chubby cheek, give them a kiss and whisper *'I love you, goodnight'* … Now imagine placing your precious child in to that moses basket for the first time and the last time, knowing it would be the very last time you see them, knowing it would be the very last time you ever get to tell your child you love them to their physical body. Ever.

Now picture: instead of your child laying in bed tonight fast asleep where they are warm and cosy – picture that child in a coffin, in the ground. A tiny blue or pink coffin, with the Earth surrounding them.

Did that hurt? Was that painful to think about? Now take that pain, multiply it a million times. Is it hurting more now? Imagine that ache. Imagine that agony. And do you know something? That STILL does not come even remotely close to describing the pain that stillbirth mummies and daddies feel.

Do you understand, now? Do you understand how utterly broken the parents of stillborn children feel? Do you understand how agonising it must be for a parent to have to imagine everything about their child and what their life would have been had they lived? Do you understand how harrowing it must have been for Chris and I to start planning our son's funeral before he had even passed away?

Please, if ever you feel the need to say/write something, not only to me but to ANY loss parent, THINK first. Think about what you are saying; think about whether what you are saying is patronising or harmful. Think about whether what you're saying will belittle the person you're saying it to.

What you probably won't know, and what many stillbirth parents won't tell you, is that even YEARS down the line, they may cry for their baby every single night. We don't just grieve for our immediate loss. We don't just grieve for the child that was. We grieve for the child that would have been.

It's been six weeks since Otis was born, and right now I'm grieving for his first smile. I will NEVER see my little boy smile, I can only imagine how perfectly cute he looks when he smiles. In 6 months or so I will be grieving for my son's first word. In a year or so, I will be grieving for my son's first steps. In 2 years or so I will be grieving for my son's first days of pre-school. In 5 years I will be grieving for my son's first day at primary school. In 11 years I will be grieving for my son's first day of secondary school. In 15/16 years I will be grieving for my son's first day of college. In around 25 years I will be grieving for my son's wedding day. In 26/27 years I will be grieving for the grandchildren I never had that he may have blessed me with…

You see, grief does not end with our loss. This is only the beginning. I will grieve for my son for the rest of my life. No, I won't cry every single day for the next 50 years or however long I live. No, I won't be moping around writing blog posts about him 2 or 3 times a day for the rest of my life. No, I won't mention him in EVERY SINGLE THING I do. Yes, I will eventually move forward. But he will always be on my mind. Otis will always be my child. He will always be the first thing I think about when I wake up, alongside Maisie and Cora; and the last thing I think about when I fall asleep, alongside Maisie and Cora.

My little boy died, his memory did not.

Otis Dominic Anthony Cullen; we miss you, we love you, we will do both eternally.

June 28th 2016.

Dear Diary,

I've spent a lot of time thinking about how Cora and Maisie have seen the events over the last few weeks unfold. I thought it may be beneficial to me to write this entry from one of their points of view... Write it as a four year old; write it as it flows. So when I read back on it, I can try and understand what I THINK may be going on in the minds of my two little girls. So, here goes...

I'm Cora, and my sister is Maisie. We are twins and we were born on the 19th of January 2012. I'm the older twin by a whole 30 seconds and boy, do I know it! Mummy and daddy aren't together, but they are friends and they get on really well, especially for me and Maisie.

Mummy tells us all the time that we are her life. That we are her strength. That we are her reason for laughing when she doesn't even feel like smiling anymore. I don't think mummy would be getting through this without the cuddles and kisses from me and Maisie.

It was hard, learning that my baby brother wasn't coming home from the hospitals with my mummy. I don't like hospitals anymore. I'm only four years old. Mummy tells me that losing our little brother is something we shouldn't have to endure – *whatever that word means.* She also tells us that she is super duper proud because we are very strong. Me and Maisie have cried a lot since Otis was born because we wanted him to come home. We didn't want to leave him in the hospital because we didn't know where he would be going next. But granddad and aunty Zoe kept telling us that everything was going to be okay, that our little brother would be looked after by Grandma Sue, Grandma Lilian and his Granny and Granddad Cullen.

Mummy can't talk about Otis to me and Maisie yet without crying, but that's okay because we can! Me and Maisie talk to each other about him all the time, especially when we think mummy can't hear us. We tell each other how much we miss him, but we say it with a smile on our face because mummy has told us that we will see him again one day, so we don't have to miss him forever and ever.

I remember Granddad first telling us when our little baby brother was poorly. It was a sad day. Mummy was crying and I heard her mutter something about it being *'inevitable that Otis will pass away.'* I'm only four, I didn't know what that meant but I knew it was sad. But I didn't cry, because I still thought my baby brother would be coming home from the hospital with mummy.

I also remember the day Otis was born. I remember grandma Ann telling us that mummy had let her know he was here. I remember her saying it expecting her to be happy, but Grandma Ann was very sad. I still didn't understand why everyone was sad about my baby brother being born. It was going to be the best! Maisie and me had even picked out his nursery theme. We wanted it to be a jungle, because Otis was going to be a little monkey.

Granddad picked us up from Grandma's house after we had our dinner. We had omelette that day, our favourite. I remember because it was after having my omelette that Granddad and aunty weewee (zoe) told us our baby brother was sleeping. *'Sleeping? Well, that's okay'* I thought, *'me and Maisie go to sleep every single night.'* But then Granddad told us he was an angel. I'd heard that before, that someone I loved had become an angel. It was my Grandma Lilian, she became an angel not that long ago. I remember now what that means. Becoming an angel means you never come home. Becoming an angel means you only get to see your family and friends when they're sleeping, because you have a special job. Mummy told me that when Grandma got the job of becoming an angel.

I know mummy was terrified when she saw me and Maisie walk through the door to meet our little baby brother. I could tell by the way she looked at me. She had 'that look', the same one she gave me when Maisie was poorly, when Milo our doggy went to doggy Heaven, and when Grandma became an angel. But this time it was worse. Mummy cried, a lot. I didn't want to leave mummy in the hospital that day. I'm only four. I didn't want to never see my baby brother again.

Mummy told me that her already broken heart broke in to a million more pieces the second she saw our happy faces that day.

When we met Otis all we saw was our little brother. We didn't pay attention to the fact he wasn't breathing, we didn't ask mummy why he was cold and why he didn't open his eyes – we just wanted to cuddle him, kiss him, touch his fingers and play with his little toes because he was so, so very cute! Mummy and her friends call Maisie the 'baby snatcher'. She loves babies. As soon as she walks in to a room with a baby, she HAS to hold that baby, she has to love on that baby and be that baby's mummy for the day. She wanted to do that with Otis too. The second Maisie saw him she NEEDED him in her arms. Maisie held our little brother lots and lots, she didn't want to let go. We stroked his little cheeks and told him how cute he is. I don't like babies that much. I prefer big girls and boys who I can talk to and play with, but I did ask to see his feet, I stroked his little toes and played with his tiny hands too. He has the cutest little hands. They were all wrinkly, like Granddads!

I remember when Otis went to Heaven. We went to the church first. Mummy told us that it would be a sad day and lots of people would cry, but that it would be okay. Granddad told us that it was okay for us to cry that day. Maisie cried, but I didn't cry. I'm only four, I didn't really know what was happening. My mummy cried lots and lots and Granddad cuddled her lots and lots. Chris did too. I remember seeing Otis' angel box being put in to the floor – mummy told us that this is how he gets to Heaven, and that when it was dark that night he would fly up to the sky. Otis isn't in that box anymore, but it stays in the ground so when he comes down to give us kisses when we are asleep he knows where to fly to. We have put lights on his grave now so he knows where he is going and doesn't get lost.

Mummy says we have been very brave since Otis was born, even though we have struggled. Me and Maisie both like to hold pictures of Otis and cuddle him while we watch TV but sometimes we miss him a lot, and this makes us cry. Mummy tries to stay strong when we cry but sometimes she struggles too, and that's okay. We know that it's okay to cry because mummy has told us. I remember going to visit Otis' grave and asking mummy and aunty weewee if I could sleep there the night. Aunty weewee told me I couldn't because I would get cold, and I cried, because then I thought Otis would get cold too. But mummy told me he has lots and lots of blankets, lots of teddies and a woolly hat to keep him warm. I cried all night and cuddled his blanky to sleep. I'm only four. I thought my little brother would be coming home.

We also have good days. Me, Maisie and mummy talk about Otis and we smile. We talk about his big elf ears and his massive toes. We don't talk about him every day though, we don't need to. We know we always think about him and that's all that matters – mummy told us that.

I know me and Maisie will always remember Otis. We will speak about him when we want to, and we say goodnight to him every single night. Otis is an angel now. He comes down at night to kiss us when we are sleeping but we aren't allowed to see him because he has special jobs to do. We are lucky to have Otis as our baby brother, even though he isn't here on Earth, and mummy tells us all the time that he is the luckiest boy who ever graced the Earth to have me and Maisie as his big sisters. This makes me happy, because I always wanted to be a good big sister to him.

We love you Otis, lots and lots.
 Love Cora Scarlett

x

Otis Dominic Anthony Cullen; We miss you, we love you, we will do both eternally.

July 3rd 2015.

Dear Diary,

I can't believe it's been a month already since Otis was born. This grief thing is such a paradox. I really want this stage of my journey to pass – I want to find my new normal and learn to live without Otis, as I know I will HAVE to eventually. But at the same time, I invite the immense hurt. I invite the unbearable pain because it makes me feel close to my son.

So how am I feeling today?

I'm going to be brutally honest in this entry, and I will remain completely unapologetic because I don't write to get people to like what I say; I write to teach people to understand the harsh reality of stillbirth, not pussyfoot around it. The more raw I am when I speak about Otis and his passing, the more truthful I'm being about how it really is.

When dealing with the loss of your baby, you deal with a completely different journey of grief to those who lose a parent, a grandparent, a friend etc … When a child dies, you don't only grieve for what they were, you grieve for what could, should and would have been had they lived. When good old Betsy passes way at 80 years old, she has a lifetime of memories behind her that her family and friends can recollect on; when 50 year old Bert passes away, yes he still has a lot of life to live, but chances are he's grown up to have a family, he's made memories with his family, his friends and siblings have had the chance to know him.

When your baby is stillborn, the only memories you have are of those during your pregnancy. I don't know what Otis would have grown to be like (though I like to imagine). I don't know if he would have been stubborn like me and his big sister Cora, cheeky like his big sister Maisie or laid back like his daddy. I don't know if he would have enjoyed playing football or doing ballet. I don't only grieve for the loss of my child, I grieve for the rest of my days I would have had with him. I grieve for his 1st birthday, his 4th birthday, his 10th and 16th birthday. I grieve for his first day of school, his first time riding a bike, his first word, his first girlfriend or boyfriend, his first EVERYTHING that some people take for granted. I grieve for his wedding day. I grieve for the birth of any grandchildren he may have blessed me with … Something you assume during pregnancy that you're going to experience.

Right now, I'm focusing on me, I'm self centered, I'm selfish … But I'm allowed to be. I've had so many people ask me how I feel, and when I respond with *'I'm hurting'* or *'I'm numb'* or *'I don't even know'*, they tend to respond with *'I know what you mean, me too.'* Really!? You do NOT know!! I understand that people are hurting, but no one is hurting more than me or even the same as me. Not Cora and Maisie, not my sister Zoe, not my dad or Chris' parents, not even Chris.

You see, what a lot of people don't understand when a child is lost through stillbirth, is that the mother of that child has grown to bond with her child, and love her child, since she saw those two lines on that pregnancy test.

I completely understand that most of the time the father is involved from day dot, too. I completely understand that people are probably thinking *'how on Earth can she say it isn't just as hard for Chris as it is for her, he lost his child too'* … Well, here it goes … I endured sickness for Otis; I coped with countless hospital stays away from Maisie and Cora for him; I insisted on my kidneys being operated on without a general anaesthetic, just coping with gas and air and a local anaesthetic, for him; I felt Otis move inside me; I felt him kick before anyone could feel him kicking on the outside; I read him bedtime stories and sang him to sleep at night; I was fiercely protective over this little being growing within me, I felt it my duty to make sure no harm came to him from the second I knew he existed … From when I found out I was carrying this precious life I fought for him; I wanted him; I loved him. I'm not saying for a second that Chris doesn't LOVE Otis as much as I, I'm not saying he doesn't miss Otis as much as I, I'm saying that losing him hasn't had as big an impact on Chris as it has me. He will happily tell you that himself.

I understand that those around me hurt, too. I am aware that Chris struggles. I know that my dad, Chris' parents, Sam, Zoe and the twins miss him and wish he was here. But nobody longs for Otis like I do. Nobody else cries themselves to sleep every single night just because they want to touch his little fingers; nobody else literally aches to feel the weight of his little body in my arms; nobody else has a breakdown on the bathroom floor every time they go to have a bath, because Otis loved to be in water during pregnancy; nobody else has changed what they eat because certain foods remind them of Otis – he loved when I ate bananas, he'd kick and go crazy, I can't eat them anymore; nobody else around me has become absolutely fucking terrified of hospitals because of me giving birth to my dead son in one of them – even harder to deal with as a sufferer of chronic illness; nobody else has become even more terrified of visiting certain friends' houses because the last time I was there we were talking about how amazing our futures would be with this little boy I was growing.

When Otis passed away inside me; when Otis' heart stopped beating; a part of me died too. And that part of me that died is never coming back.

People tell me that I will 'move on' … Let me tell you that I will NEVER move on from the death of my son and if you don't understand why, then count your blessings. I will move forward, eventually. I will learn to live with his absence and find a new 'normal' without him here because I HAVE to. I know, deep down, if I didn't have Cora and Maisie to stay strong for, then right now I'd probably be telling you a completely different story. I am broken. My heart is shattered. I will NEVER be the same again.

So when I tell you that I'm hurting or when I tell you that I'm numb or if I tell you some days that I just don't know how I feel, please don't just tell me that you know because you feel it too. Tell me that it's okay for me to feel that way. Tell me that you sympathise but can't empathise, because you don't know what this feels like and I hope to God you never will. Tell me that it's going to become bareable, but do not tell me that it's going to be okay. It is never going to be okay that my little boy is buried in a tiny blue coffin in the ground instead of being led sleeping in his moses basket beside me.

Otis' death has changed me. He took most of me with him.

July 4th 2016.

Dear Diary,

Feeling pretty guilty today. Grandparents are so often overlooked when it comes to losing a child through stillbirth. No one seems to ever pay attention to how the mothers and fathers of mothers and fathers who lose their baby really feel. It wasn't until recently that I did myself. I got in bed one evening and just thought to myself *'it must hurt them so much, too'* … Not only are Grandparents grieving for the loss of their grandchild, they are grieving for the loss their child has to endure – just like I grieve for Maisie and Cora for losing their little brother.

One of my biggest regrets after losing Otis was not involving Chris' parents (Bernard and Thelma) more in my pregnancy. My family were 'lucky' in a sense that they were involved in Otis' life from day dot. From the day Chris and I saw those two lines on that pregnancy test, my family had our little boy in their lives. My sister and dad came to scans that Chris couldn't attend – Zoe had the opportunity to see Otis moving and seeing his little heart beating … Something that Bernard and Thelma will never get the chance to do. I will forever feel guilty for ASSUMING that our little boy would be born alive. I will forever feel guilty for taking for granted our son's heart beat and ASSUMING it would stay. I will forever feel guilty for ASSUMING that they weren't too interested in being involved in the pregnancy. I will forever feel guilty for ASSUMING they didn't want to come shopping for baby clothes, or to help me decorate his nursery. I would give anything to turn back time and invite them both to an ultrasound scan to see their little grandson alive and moving; to give them the opportunity to feel him move and kick in my tummy …

Hindsight is a beautiful thing, isn't it?

'All I can tell you is that I have been completely heartbroken since his death. I have never, ever felt such a sense of loss and helplessness as I have felt about Otis. I will hear a line in a song or see his picture (he is my phone home screen) & I'm off. And I truly don't know why. I never got to hear him cry, see him smile, change a nappy & yet I feel such an affinity with him. I'm in floods now just writing this. I was raised catholic & I attended mass, but I have not set foot in a church since his funeral. If there is a God how did he let this happen? We are not bad people. **Heartbroken.** *That is the 1 word that describes how I feel.'* – Bernard (Otis' Grandad).

I know now that, they too, feel heartbroken.
 I know now that, they too, feel an indescribable sense of loss.
 I know now that, they too, would give their very last breath to see Otis take his first.
 I know now that, they too, though differently to Chris and I, will forever mourn the loss of Otis.

Losing Otis has been the single, most devastating event that has ever, EVER happened to me. I could not imagine losing a grandchild but then also having to do my best to stay strong to support my child who needs me. I could not imagine having to watch my child suffer the way my dad has to watch me suffer, the way that Bernard and Thelma have to watch Chris suffer. I could not imagine the pain of having to stand and watch my child bury their child. I could not imagine Bernard and Thelma's agony in seeing their son carry their first grandson – their first grandchild – into the church in his coffin. I could not imagine my dad's pain in watching me break down and having to try and support me. I could not imagine my dad's pain in knowing that he could do nothing at all to change what had happened. I could not imagine the pain of losing a grandchild. And I truly hope I never do.

Admittedly, out of all of the posts I have written for my blog, this has been the hardest one. Trying to empathise with my dad, Bernard and Thelma is hard – putting myself in their shoes and seeing this tragedy from their point of view; it really fucking hurts.

I've been selfish. All I have thought about since Otis died is myself and how I feel; all I have focused on is my grief and the girls' grief. I didn't once stop to ask my dad if he is okay. I didn't once send a text or a mail to either of Chris' parents asking them how they are coping. Not only am I realising as I write this that I've deprived Otis' Grandparents of knowing their grandchild alive; I have also ignored their mourning.

I will be forever sorry for that.

One thing I made sure happened when Otis was born, was that his grandparents got to meet him. If anything, I pushed it. I knew it was the only one chance they were ever going to get to see their precious grandson in the flesh.

As soon as my dad walked in to the delivery suite when I had given birth, I saw the love he had for Otis in his eyes, but the sadness that he wasn't here. It was the most bittersweet moment. My dad spoke to Otis just as he would have had he been born alive; he spoke to me about how surprised he was with his weight and length (we were told to expect him to be small as he had stopped growing); he even joked with me and Nicola (our midwife) about how well endowed he was! It was my dad and my step mum, Sam, talking to and about Otis the way they did and do that made me realise it was okay to enjoy the good times too. It is okay not to be 100% sad and incapable of speaking happy things about my little boy. It was my dad and Sam who taught me that I was allowed to be happy he existed; I was allowed to be happy that he did once have a heartbeat, even if he didn't anymore; I was allowed to speak about what could, should and would have been had Otis been born alive. It was my dad and Sam who taught me that, one day, I will speak about Otis with a smile instead of tears in my eyes, and that this is completely okay. It is my dad and Sam who have taught me that I don't have to carry this overwhelming feeling of grief, guilt and regret with me for the rest of my life. They have done all this without even speaking those words, just through their actions I have learned that I can find happiness again. I can love fully again. And in time, I will.

I cannot put in to words how grateful I am for the both of them.

I will always have imprinted on my mind the moment that Chris' mum and dad walked in to the room to meet their grandson. Their apprehension in meeting him, their nervousness in seeing Chris and I … The second they laid eyes on Otis they fell in love. I could see it just by looking at them; I could see the love they had (and still have) for Otis in the tears falling from their cheeks. I could see the fear they felt in holding him because he was so perfectly fragile. I could see the admiration they had for our little boy's beauty. I could see the helplessness they felt that there was nothing they could do for Otis, Chris and myself.

Otis really does have the most amazing grandparents. Grandparents who will honour him for the rest of their days. Grandparents who will speak of him and involve him in everything they do. Grandparents that are PROUD he existed and fought so hard to meet them. Grandparents that will treasure every single picture they have of him. Grandparents who LOVE him in death as much as they would have in life.

Thank you, dad. Thank you, Sam. Thank you, Bernard. Thank you, Thelma. Thank you for being all you have been and doing all you do for Chris and I. There are no words in existence to explain how much I appreciate you all.

'Moments in time that should have been filled with our joy are forever filled with our grief.' – Bernard.

July 6th 2016.

Dear Diary,

Over the last few days I have grappled with a constant niggling at the back of my mind that I need to do something about the loss that others around me are feeling due to losing Otis. I have been considering talking to Chris' parents to see if they would like to become a part of Cora and Maisie's lives (Chris is not their daddy)– not to take over, not as their 'grandparents' … Just as two people, who would grow to love them like everyone else does who meets them; who would see their precious grandson in them. Maisie and Cora's daddy's family are involved in Otis' life in the sense of keeping his memory alive, and they often spoke of how he would be as much in their lives as the girls. They even came to Otis' funeral … I'm happy, in that sense, that I have children with two of the most caring families I know.

Had Otis lived, they would have grown to know the girls through seeing them at birthday parties etc, and I didn't want our future lives to do a complete turnaround and change because he's no longer here. I don't think that Otis would want for two families NOT to become one just because he isn't here. I don't think Otis would want for everyone just to walk their separate ways because then life wouldn't be as it would if he was living. Everything would be different. A massive part of me wants life, in that sense, to carry on as it would had he lived, because then I would feel as though I'm honouring his memory.

I thought, after the last few weeks and losing Otis, that the girls would offer Chris' parents some peace. They are the nearest anyone has to Otis. They share 50% of their DNA with our little boy – something that no one else in the world does apart from his daddy and I. I wanted to see if it would provide them some comfort after losing Otis. I went to bed confused with this thought on my mind, not knowing what to do, not knowing if I should ask, not knowing how anyone would react if I suggested it... You could say I felt stupid, and scared, for even thinking it. But it gave me some hope. It gave me hope that Chris' parents would be able to enjoy the girls as Otis' siblings. It gave me hope that the girls would help Chris' parents see who their little grandson would have been had he been born alive.

They would get to know how funny Maisie is; how, regardless of the situation, she is always there to help other people. They would get to know how much Maisie would have mothered Otis and how loved on he would have been by her. They would get to know how intelligent Cora is and how she likes to teach others. They would get to see how much Otis would have learned from his big sister, Cora. They would also get to see just how stubborn she is! From getting to know the girls, they would get to know a part of their grandson, too. Whether that would be a reassuring and comforting thing, or the complete opposite and make them miss him more, is something we wouldn't know the answer to until it happened.

Anyway, last night, I had a dream. In my dream they must have accepted my invitation for them to meet the twins and become a part of their lives. We were all on a beach, not sure which one or where, but it was a beautiful beach with the whitest sand and the bluest sea I have ever seen. There was no clouds in sight and the sun was beaming. Bernard and Thelma (Chris' mum and dad) were further up the beach playing with Maisie and Cora, while I sat watching them. I remember feeling a little at peace – something I haven't felt at all since Otis passed away. It felt good, but wrong at the same time.

In my dream, I turned to the left of me for just a second because I heard a noise. I caught a glimpse of this child playing in the distance, with no adult with them. I had a quick glimpse around the beach to see if I could spot any adults that could be supervising – there were none. I took it upon myself to walk up this child and see if they were okay, and if they had anyone with them.

As I was walking over, this child turned to look at me. It was a little boy and he was absolutely beautiful! He had the biggest blue eyes, dark hair (and a lot of it) and a cute button nose. He just looked up at me and said *'I'm okay. It's okay. I know that I'm loved.'* At this point I was really confused and told him that we would go and find his mummy. He replied *'okay.'* I turned back to Bernard and Thelma to tell them I was going to take this little boy back to his parents. With a confused look on their faces they asked me *'what little boy? There's no one there.'* The beach was completely empty.

Shaking off what had just happened I started walking back to where I was sat, then out of the corner of my eye I saw him again, he was walking in to the water. How could I see this little boy, but no one else could?

Then I saw him look at me. I looked back at him. For a moment, time stood still. It was then that I realised this little boy was MY little boy. It was my son. It was Otis.

(I get goosebumps as I write this)

I had realised that this beautiful little being was my son after he had grown up a little. His eyes were open, and they were stunning! He could walk, he could talk, he could BREATHE by himself – something the doctors told us Otis would never do. He wasn't riddled by brain tumour, his body wasn't riddled with haemorrhages, he wasn't showing any signs of pain. Heaven must have taken all that away from him. In my dream, he was happy, he was free. In my dream he KNEW how loved he is!

A part of me now thinks that this (in some strange way) was my subconscious letting me know that whatever I felt I had to do, was okay to do. It was like my mind was telling me that, regardless of what happens in the future, I will never replace Otis and he knows that I would never replace him. Another part of me also thinks that it was my brain's way of letting me know that I don't have to worry about Otis (though I always will) because wherever he may be now, he can see. He can see the world he couldn't see when he was with us. He can watch his big sisters play. He can watch his mummy, daddy, grandparents, aunts and uncles LOVE him from afar. He can do anything he wants to do and be anything he wants to be, because there are no limits in Heaven.

Whether I truly believe there is a Heaven or not, I don't know – only time will tell. I don't know whether I believe it because I genuinely think there is one, or as a comfort that my little boy isn't just rotting in his tiny blue coffin in the ground. I HAVE to believe that his soul, his entity, is somewhere other than that coffin. I HAVE to believe in something or I wouldn't be coping.

After having that dream, I'm reassured that everyone around me (and Otis) know that I would never, ever consider trying to replace my son in anyone's lives. I am reassured that it's okay to do what I feel I need to do to get through losing him, and help others around me get through losing him. We will NEVER move on, but I'm reassured it's okay to eventually move forward. I'm reassured that it's okay to try and see Otis in other people and that it's 'normal' to feel guilty for doing so.

Otis Dominic Anthony Cullen; We love you, we miss you, we will do both eternally.

<u>**July 9th 2016.**</u>

Dear Diary,

I'm fuming!

I've been very open about Otis and his death since we left the hospital on the 5th of June. Not only because he didn't grace the Earth to die in vain; I didn't want him to be another baby forgotten because he DIED in utero and that's a taboo subject.

I chose to share Otis and his story because I refuse to let my little boy become part of a statistic.

When you become a mummy, it becomes your duty to protect your child.
When you become a mummy and your child dies, it becomes your duty to protect your child's memory.

Stillbirth is the unspoken word of pregnancy. It's a statistic. It's taboo. It's a stigma. It's also reality. Not once through my pregnancy was I told "stillbirth happens" or made aware of how OFTEN stillbirth happens. In this day and age, with the access we have to technology, it should not be happening.

A 'stillborn' baby defines a baby born with no heartbeat over 24 weeks of gestation. Over 3500 babies are stillborn every year in the UK. A lot of people associate these babies with having something wrong with them when, in reality, only 1 in 10 babies that are stillborn have a genetic abnormality or serious condition that prevents them from living a full life or being completely incompatible with life. *How SCARY is that?* 9 out of 10 babies that pass away in utero do so for *"no reason"* … due to *"tragic accident"* (starvation of oxygen, blood clots getting in to the umbilical cord etc).

Stillbirth needs to be spoken about. This is the reason I am sharing our story.

Before Otis I was more than ignorant to stillbirth myself, because I never expected it to happen to me. I was aware of it, I knew what it was, but I didn't know at all what it entailed and I certainly didn't know just how common it is.

Since sharing Otis' story I have had people come forward telling me how thankful they are and how much they appreciate me speaking up on Facebook etc. I've had numerous people tell me that it's thanks to me and Otis they now have the strength to share their stories too.

That was lovely. My mom had a still birth when I was 3ish and I don't remember anything about that time. Reading your posts and, especially this blog post, make me curious about my reaction at that time. It is encouraging me to have a conversation with my mom about that time in our lives. Thank you for that. – Amanda.

I always hesitated to read your blog before because it does bring back memories of my twins but something made me read this one and I had to say thank you! Reading this was hard yes not a dry eye here but i needed that... It's ok to not be ok sometimes... I'm happy to see your girls are doing ok through this experience. Huge hugs. – Martine.

Beautiful! I had a stillbirth in November. At that time my older boys were 18 months and 3. And I have to agree my heart broke into a million more pieces, too, when my 3 year old asked why I didn't bring his baby sister home. 8 months later, he still talks about her being in heaven. I always wonder if it's something he will remember or just fade away. As I was sent far away to a specialty hospital to deliver and the boys never got to meet her. I guess time will tell. Thank you for Sharing. It makes it more comfortable to talk about what happened to us in November. – Tanisha.

That was beautiful. Reminded me a lot of how I felt when my own brother didn't come home from the hospital. I'm so glad your girls got to see him, I truly believe it will make all of the difference in their lives. I know I wish I had. Thank you for using your experience in such a powerful positive way. Hugs to you from across the pond. – Danielle.

Those messages, right there, are why I am doing what I do.

Since I started sharing our journey of grief, countless men and women – mummies and daddies – have told me about their journey with stillbirth; each one harrowing, each one different to the next. I'm happy people trust me to share, I'm happy people find the courage to share, but it frustrates me that there are so many people in the same situation as me. It upsets me knowing there are so many people who only have a gravestone or a tub of ashes to look at when they speak to their child. I hate knowing that there were so many people before me who know this pain, and I hate even more, now knowing what this pain feels like, that there are so many people after me who will know this pain.

So for those who insist on believing that I am sharing Otis' story purely for attention, please know that you could not be more wrong. I would give the world to be sharing stories about my 1 month old baby and how he would just be learning to smile for the first time. I would give the world to be sharing pictures of my growing boy. I would give the world to have announced to the world that my 5lbs1oz bundle of pure perfection was born crying. I would give the world to see my son with his eyes open, even just the once. I would give my very last breath, just to see Otis take his first.

Every single time I write about Otis my heart breaks, it takes a LOT out of me to do this. It is mentally and emotionally exhausting, forcing myself to remember every last feeling and every last memory that another part of me is trying to force myself to forget and move forward from. Every time I write about Otis, I grieve that bit more for what should, could and would have been. Every time I write about Otis, I get a small realisation that my little boy is dead, adding to the bigger realisation that my little boy is NEVER coming home. I don't do this for me. I do this for Otis, and the 3500+ other babies born with *no voice*.

July 10th 2016.

Dear Diary,

One of the most difficult things in the world to do after losing a child, is to carry on being a good mum to the ones I have earth side. Not because I'm not capable, but because I'm worried about smothering them through fear. It's hard to let them leave my sight for fear of losing them too, but I have to. It's hard to let them do anything that could hurt them, even if it's just running around knowing they can trip and fall, ...but I have to. I don't know how I'm going to cope come September when they start school full time.

My single biggest fear has always been losing a child, but I always deemed it irrational, convincing myself it would never happen to me. It has happened to me, so that fear has now become completely rational and I am beyond terrified it will happen again. I don't want to bury any more children. This is another reality of stillbirth - the fear it instils in to you for the rest of your life

July 12th 2016

Dear Diary,

Since losing Otis, not only have we grappled with agonising grief, but also comments off those around us (and even strangers) that just do not help our situation. I know that people don't make such comments to purposely upset us and I also know their heart is USUALLY in the right place (some people are just downright nasty), but there are some things that just don't need to be said to a bereaved parent – things people would never find appropriate to say to people when their grandparent, parent, sibling, uncle, aunty, and so on, pass away.

"God needed another angel." Really?! He did?! I NEEDED my son more!

" At least you have other children at home." Please, tell me which of your children you would choose to give back? Tell me which of your children you would choose to organise a funeral for instead of a birthday party? Tell me which of your children you can live without? YES, I have the girls, that does not make my little boy any less loved, any less wanted or any less missed than what he would be if they weren't here.

" God only gives you what you can handle." What about what I deserve? I know I have made mistakes in my life but I have always and will always do my best by my children. I didn't deserve

for my son to die, whether I am apparently strong enough to cope with it or not. And how do you know I can 'handle' this? If you must know, I spend my nights crying myself to sleep, and I only manage to sleep through pure exhaustion. Every time I close my eyes I see Otis, I see him being placed on to my chest for the first time and realising that the doctors were right, that he wasn't alive. Every time I close my eyes I imagine what my life would be like and how different it would be if my little boy was here. Every time I close my eyes I think to myself *'I should be being woken up by a crying baby needing comfort from his mummy'*. I am NOT strong, I can NOT handle this. I cope for the girls because I have no choice.

"I know how you feel." This is the worst one for me. Unless you have given birth to a fully formed baby with no heartbeat, unless you have planned a funeral for one of your children, unless you have sat with a doctor or midwife and heard those soul destroying words *'I'm sorry, there's no heartbeat'* do NOT tell me you know how I feel. Do you know how it feels to dress your child in to their second ever outfit, and their last? Do you know how it feels knowing that your child only has a second outfit because you want to take the first home, just to remind you of their size and smell? Do you know how it feels to dress your child in to their burial outfit instead of their coming home outfit? Do you know how it feels to go through an agonising labour to push out your cold, still, silent baby? Unless you do, do NOT tell me you know how I feel, because you don't and I hope you never, ever do. I would not wish this pain on my worst enemy, so please do not wish it upon yourself by saying you know how this feels.

"At least you can have another baby." Forgive me, are you a doctor now? How do you know this? What a lot of people don't know, is that the condition that caused Otis' death is genetic and it is VERY possible the same could happen again if I ever had another baby. I got stupidly lucky with the girls, like winning the lottery twice. When people say this it feels like they are telling you your child is replaceable, that when you have another baby you will suddenly 'get over' and forget that your child ever existed. I will think of my little boy for the rest of my life, I will move forward and I will learn to live without him, but I will never move on whether I do have another baby in the future or not.

"I'm here for you." Please, do not say this to a bereaved parent unless you actually intend on being there for them. SO many people have told this since losing Otis. A lot of people wrote statuses on Facebook the day they found out our little boy passed away saying it, but have never once privately acknowledged me. It's like people want the world to know they are a part of this situation, when in reality they really aren't – for a bit of sympathy, I guess. People who hadn't spoken to me throughout my entire pregnancy suddenly became 'friends' again when they found out Otis had passed away, and I've taken it upon myself to not let these 'friends' back in my life. Selfish maybe, but this is the one time in my life I have every right to be selfish and protect myself.

"He's in a better place." NO, no he is not! The best place for my son is in mine and his daddy's arms. The best place for my son is here, on Earth, with his big sisters.

"I'm sorry." Why? What are you sorry for? This is something that should, in theory, be comforting to parents, but for me and many angel parents around me, it feels awkward. What am I supposed to respond when you tell me you're sorry? I've actually found myself saying *'that's okay, it isn't your fault'*. I am not sorry that Otis was born, and I haven't met one bereaved parent who has said otherwise about their child. The only thing I'm sorry for is that Otis never got to stay. I 100% believe there was a reason he fought so hard to live, and I am determined to find that reason and honour it for him.

Otis Dominic Anthony Cullen; We miss you, we love you, we will do both eternally.

July 15th 2016.

Dear Diary,

I think I'm starting to struggle a little. I want my son back.

I did not deserve this. Nor did his daddy. His sisters definitely didn't. His Grandma and Grandad Cullen didn't deserve to lose their first grandson – their first grandchild. My dad and Sam didn't deserve to lose their grandson. My little brother didn't deserve to lose his playmate and nephew. My sisters didn't deserve to lose their nephew. Chris' brother and his fiancée didn't deserve to lose their nephew. Our friends didn't deserve to lose their childrens' playmate … I'm annoying myself saying that, because we didn't 'lose' him. We didn't take him to Mothercare shopping for his baby clothes and leave him there, we didn't forget to bring him home from the hospital. We haven't LOST him. He's dead. He's gone. Forever. Never coming back. I won't ever feel his skin again, I won't ever cuddle him again, I won't ever kiss his little face again. I won't ever see him in his daddy's arms again. I won't ever see his grandparents love on him again. Ever.

Otis is one of the most loved little boys who ever graced the Earth; he would have had an amazing life. He'd be a month old now and just learning to smile, just learning to focus his eyes on the people whose voices he had heard but couldn't quite make out their faces yet …

This is is not fair.

Chris and I would give our very last breath just to see our son have his first.

I want my son back.

Otis Dominic Anthony Cullen; we miss you, we love you, we will do both eternally.

<u>**July 16th 2016.**</u>

Dear Diary,

I really hope this pain starts to ease. I cannot cope with it anymore.

Please, please tell me it gets better.

www.ingramcontent.com/pod-product-compliance
Lightning Source LLC
Chambersburg PA
CBHW052015280526
45793CB00005B/986